PULSE
Emergency Ultrasound Guide

PULSE
Emergency Ultrasound Guide

Editor-in-Chief

Alka Verma
MD FACEE
Additional Professor
Department of Emergency Medicine
Sanjay Gandhi Postgraduate Institute of Medical Sciences
Lucknow, Uttar Pradesh, India

Editors

Divya Srivastava
MD PDCC FACEE MAMS
Additional Professor
Department of Anesthesiology
Sanjay Gandhi Postgraduate Institute of Medical Sciences
Lucknow, Uttar Pradesh, India

Subhankar Paul
MD DrNB FCCU
Senior Consultant
Department of Critical Care Medicine
Medanta Super Speciality Hospital
Lucknow, Uttar Pradesh, India

Lokendra Gupta
MBBS MD DNB (CCM) MRCEM (UK)
Director (Emergency Medicine and Trauma Care)
Medanta Super Speciality Hospital
Lucknow, Uttar Pradesh, India

Forewords

Slaven Bajic
Thiagarajan Jaiganesh
Hari Govind Sukumaran

JAYPEE

JAYPEE BROTHERS MEDICAL PUBLISHERS
The Health Sciences Publisher
New Delhi | London

Jaypee Brothers Medical Publishers (P) Ltd

Headquarters
EMCA House, 23/23-B
Ansari Road, Daryaganj
New Delhi 110 002, India
Landline: +91-11-23272143, +91-11-23272703
+91-11-23282021, +91-11-23245672
e-mail: jaypee@jaypeebrothers.com

Corporate Office
4838/24, Ansari Road, Daryaganj
New Delhi 110 002, India
Phone: +91-11-43574357
Fax: +91-11-43574314
e-mail: jaypee@jaypeebrothers.com

Overseas Office
JP Medical Ltd
83 Victoria Street, London
SW1H 0HW (UK)
Phone: +44-20 3170 8910
e-mail: info@jpmedpub.com

EU GPSR Authorised Representative
Logos Europe, 9 rue Nicolas Poussin
17000, La Rochelle, France
Phone: +33 (0) 6 67 93 73 78
e-mail: contact@logoseurope.eu

Website: www.jaypeebrothers.com
Website: www.jaypeedigital.com

Inquiries for bulk sales may be solicited at: jaypee@jaypeebrothers.com

PULSE Emergency Ultrasound Guide

First Edition: **2026**

ISBN: 978-93-7202-926-0

Printed at: Samrat Offset Pvt. Ltd.

Contributors

Alka Verma MD FACEE
Additional Professor
Department of Emergency Medicine
Sanjay Gandhi Postgraduate Institute of Medical Sciences
Lucknow, Uttar Pradesh, India

Amit Anand MD DM
Assistant Professor
Department of Medicine and Cardiac Intensive Unit
King George's Medical University
Lucknow, Uttar Pradesh, India

Ashish Kumar Kannaujia MD
Professor
Department of Anesthesia
Sanjay Gandhi Postgraduate Institute of Medical Sciences
Lucknow, Uttar Pradesh, India

Asif Dabeer Jafri MD MRCP (UK) MRCPI MRCPE DEM
Senior Registrar
Department of Emergency Medicine
Sanjay Gandhi Postgraduate Institute of Medical Sciences
Lucknow, Uttar Pradesh, India

Chetna Shamshery MD DNB PDCC MNAMS
Additional Professor
Department of Anesthesiology
Sanjay Gandhi Postgraduate Institute of Medical Sciences
Lucknow, Uttar Pradesh, India

Divya Srivastava
MD PDCC FACEE MAMS
Additional Professor
Department of Anesthesiology
Sanjay Gandhi Postgraduate Institute of Medical Sciences
Lucknow, Uttar Pradesh, India

Harshit Agarwal MBBS MS MCh
Senior Consultant
Department of Trauma Surgery and Critical Care
Shri Ram Murti Smarak Institute of Medical Sciences
Bareilly, Uttar Pradesh, India

Lokendra Gupta
MBBS MD DNB (CCM) MRCEM (UK)
Director (Emergency Medicine and Trauma Care)
Medanta Super Speciality Hospital
Lucknow, Uttar Pradesh, India

Nidhi Singh DM DrNB
Assistant Professor
Department of Anesthesiology
Sanjay Gandhi Postgraduate Institute of Medical Sciences
Lucknow, Uttar Pradesh, India

Pallav Singh MD PDAF
Assistant Professor
Department of Anesthesiology
Sanjay Gandhi Postgraduate Institute of Medical Sciences
Lucknow, Uttar Pradesh, India

Pooja Gautam MD
Senior Resident
Department of Emergency Medicine
Sanjay Gandhi Postgraduate Institute of Medical Sciences
Lucknow, Uttar Pradesh, India

Prem Raj Singh MD
Professor (Jr Grade)
Department of Anesthesia and Critical Care
King George's Medical University
Lucknow, Uttar Pradesh, India

Pushpraj Singh MD PDCC FISC
Senior Consultant
Department of Critical Care Medicine
Charak Hospital and Research Centre
Lucknow, Uttar Pradesh, India

Ruchi Verma MD PDCC MAMS
Additional Professor
Department of Anesthesiology
Sanjay Gandhi Postgraduate Institute of Medical Sciences
Lucknow, Uttar Pradesh, India

Shefali Gautam MD
Professor (Jr Grade)
Department of Anesthesia and Critical Care
King George's Medical University
Lucknow, Uttar Pradesh, India

Shyam Sundar MD DNB PDCC
PGDUS Fellowship in Cardiology
Senior Resident
Department of Emergency Medicine
Sanjay Gandhi Postgraduate Institute of Medical Sciences
Lucknow, Uttar Pradesh, India

Subhankar Paul MD DrNB FCCU
Senior Consultant
Department of Critical Care Medicine
Medanta Super Speciality Hospital
Lucknow, Uttar Pradesh, India

Suruchi Ambasta MBBS MD
Associate Professor
Department of Anesthesiology
Sanjay Gandhi Postgraduate Institute of Medical Sciences
Lucknow, Uttar Pradesh, India

Utsav Anand Mani MD
Assistant Professor
Department of Emergency Medicine
Sanjay Gandhi Postgraduate Institute of Medical Sciences
Lucknow, Uttar Pradesh, India

Vijeta Bajpai MBBS MD
Associate Professor
Department of Anesthesiology, Pain Medicine and Critical Care
All India Institute of Medical Sciences
Gorakhpur, Uttar Pradesh, India

Foreword

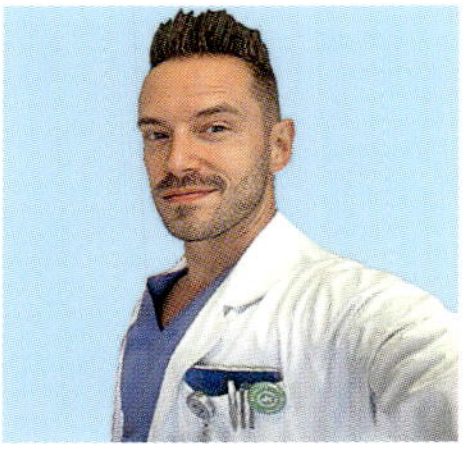

Point-of-care ultrasound (POCUS) has become an essential tool in emergency medicine today. While we once referred to POCUS as the stethoscope of the future, the truth is—it has become the stethoscope of the present!

POCUS is now a fundamental tool in the hands of emergency physicians worldwide. Whether used at the bedside in a busy hospital emergency department or on the roadside during a trauma call, its ability to provide real-time, dynamic, and life-saving information is unparalleled. In environments where access to X-ray, CT, or advanced diagnostics is limited—or entirely absent—POCUS becomes not only useful, but also indispensable.

From urban hospitals to rural clinics, from disaster zones to combat operations, and from ambulance teams to air evacuation units, POCUS allows clinicians to make faster, safer, and more accurate decisions. Its role in guiding procedures, assessing critical patients, and answering focused clinical questions cannot be overstated.

In India, where healthcare delivery often spans a vast range of environments—from world-class tertiary centers to underserved rural regions—the value of POCUS is particularly profound. Its portability, cost-effectiveness, and diagnostic power make it an ideal technology to bridge healthcare gaps and enhance patient outcomes across the spectrum of care.

I strongly encourage all young emergency medicine doctors—and any clinician working in acute care settings—to pursue formal education and continuous training in POCUS. Mastery of this tool not only enhances diagnostic capability but also sharpens clinical thinking, strengthens procedural safety, and ultimately saves lives.

This manual is a timely and valuable contribution to POCUS education. It represents a practical guide for integrating ultrasound into everyday clinical practice, regardless of setting. Whether you are just beginning your journey with ultrasound or looking to refine your existing skills, I believe this resource will become a trusted companion in your professional development.

POCUS is no longer optional—it is a standard of care. Learn it, use it, and never stop improving!

Slaven Bajic MD
Emergency Medicine Specialist, MCoROM
Izola General Hospital, Slovenia, EU
POCUS US instructor for EUSEM, Winfocus and COROM

Foreword

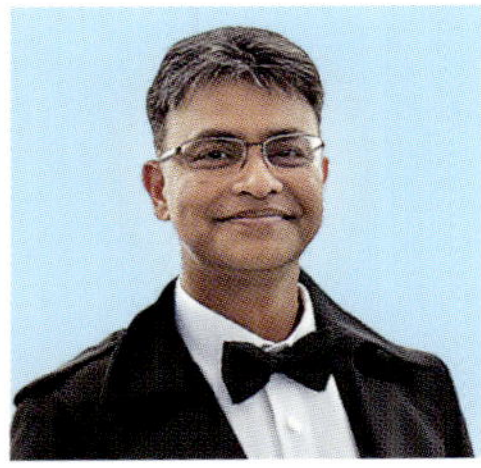

Emergency medicine has always thrived at the intersection of urgency and innovation. Few tools have demonstrated such transformative impact at the bedside as ultrasound. Its ability to provide immediate, dynamic insights in the heat of critical care has changed the way we diagnose, intervene, and save lives.

PULSE: Emergency Ultrasound Guide is a timely and vital contribution to this evolving landscape. *PULSE—Proactive Ultrasound in Life-Saving Emergencies*—is more than a clever acronym; it is a philosophy of practice. It reflects the belief that ultrasound is not simply an adjunct to care but a core clinical instrument—an extension of the physician's eyes and hands in the most time-sensitive settings.

What distinguishes this guide is its comprehensive scope and practical clarity. It addresses not just the basics of machine handling and "knobology," but extends into specialized domains—neuro, airway, lung, cardiac, abdominal, vascular, musculoskeletal, and procedural ultrasound—culminating in structured approaches to cardiac arrest scenarios. Each module is anchored in clinical reality, offering both the "why" and the "how" of ultrasound use. By distilling complex science into clear protocols—such as the SESAME, BLUE, and FALLS frameworks—this guide enables rapid, reproducible, and lifesaving decision-making.

The urgency of this work cannot be overstated. Portable ultrasound machines are now widely available, but their impact is blunted if training, application, and protocols remain inconsistent. It is, therefore, the need of the hour to standardize the role of ultrasound in every emergency department (ED) so that a patient in one ED receives the same quality of care as a patient in another. The PULSE course and methodology presented here can serve as a uniform standard protocol, bridging gaps in practice, reducing variability, and enhancing patient safety.

As educators, we know that knowledge without structure remains underutilized. What this book achieves is the creation of an algorithm-based, protocol-driven approach that can be taught, mastered, and sustained across all levels of emergency care. It turns ultrasound from an occasional convenience into a routine necessity.

I commend the authors for this monumental effort. This guide is not only a teaching resource; it is a call to action—for departments, institutions, and systems to embrace ultrasound as an indispensable pillar of emergency medicine. If widely adopted, PULSE has the potential to redefine standards of care, streamline emergency responses, and, most importantly, save countless lives.

May this book serve as both a guide and a movement, empowering physicians to scan, spot, and save—proactively, consistently, and universally.

Thiagarajan Jaiganesh
FRCS (Surg) FRCS (A/E) FRCEM CMQ MBA
Chairman, Emergency Department
STMC, Tawam & Al Ain Hospitals
Consultant, Adult and Pediatric Emergency Medicine
Former Program Director, Tawam EM Residency (2016–2023)
Adjunct Assistant, UAE University

Foreword

PULSE: The Clinician's Imperative

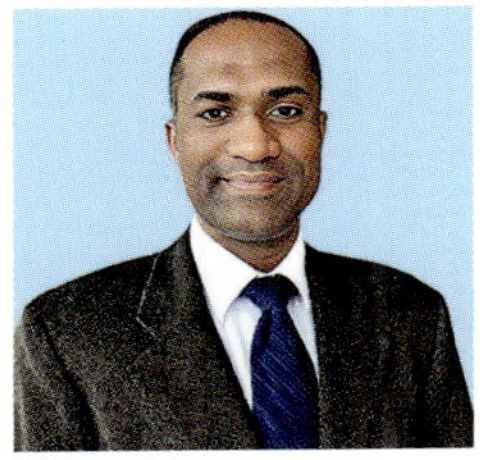

For decades, the art of emergency medicine has been defined by speed, precision, and an unwavering commitment to patient care at the bedside. The stethoscope was our symbol and the X-ray, our first window into the unknown. But a new era has arrived. Point-of-care ultrasound (POCUS) is no longer the "stethoscope of the future"—it is the present standard, fundamentally altering the diagnostic and procedural paradigm for every senior emergency physician.

This is a shift not of technology, but of philosophy. POCUS empowers us to transcend the limitations of traditional physical examinations, providing real-time, dynamic, and actionable insight into the most time-critical conditions. Whether in the chaos of a busy resuscitation bay, the isolation of a prehospital scene, or the res006Furce-limited environment of a humanitarian mission, ultrasound is the definitive extension of our clinical acumen.

From rapidly narrowing a complex differential diagnosis to guiding life-saving procedures with unmatched precision, POCUS has redefined what is possible at the bedside. Its immediacy, versatility, and portability make it uniquely suited to every challenge we face, enabling us to deliver the highest standard of care when every second counts.

This guide, *PULSE: Emergency Ultrasound Guide*, is an invitation to mastery. It is an authoritative, evidence-based, and clinically focused resource designed to honor your experience while challenging you to elevate your practice. It is a roadmap to harnessing the full power of emergency ultrasound—to build on a lifetime of expertise, sharpen your diagnostic vision, and enhance the safety of your procedures.

This is more than a book. It is a call to action. POCUS is not just a skill to be learned; it is a mindset to be adopted. Embrace it and let it redefine your legacy in emergency medicine.

Hari Govind Sukumaran MD FRCEM MCEM
Clinical Director and Emergency Medicine Consultant
Emergency Department
Al Qassimi and Al Qassimi Women's and Children Hospital
Sharjah, UAE

Preface

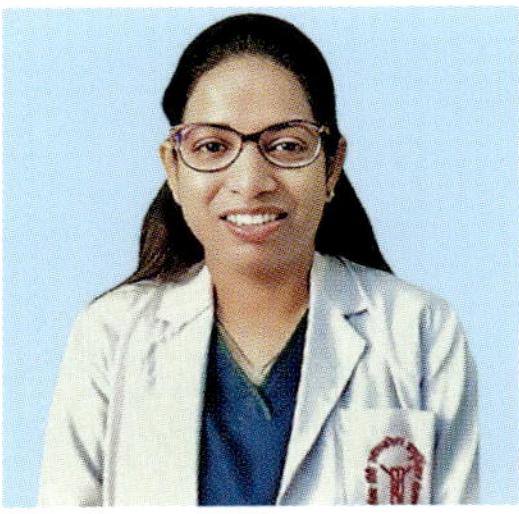

Alka Verma

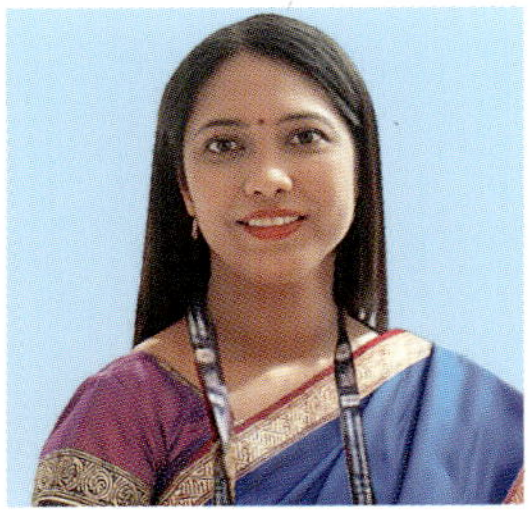

Divya Srivastava

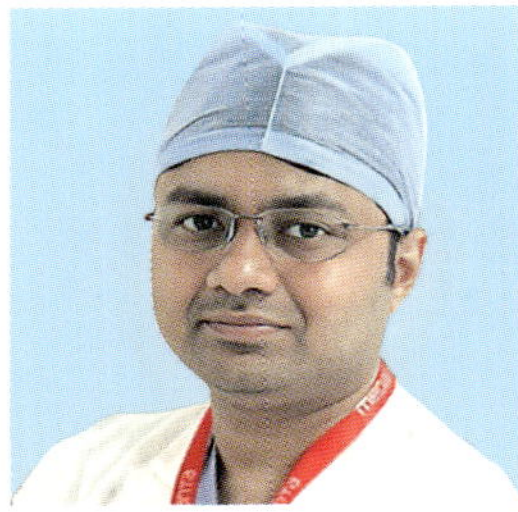

Subhankar Paul

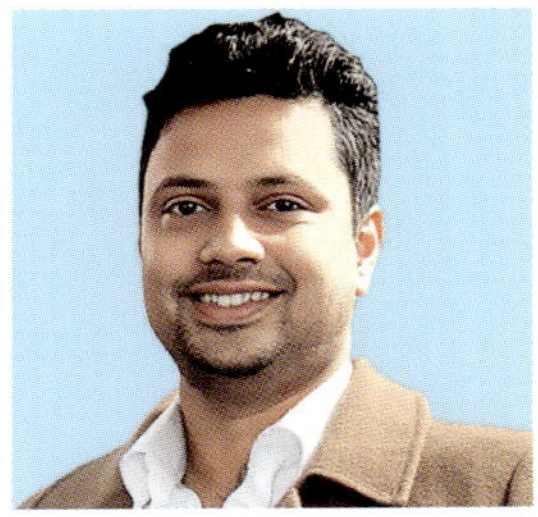

Lokendra Gupta

The field of ultrasonography has undergone a profound transformation in recent years. What was once the exclusive domain of radiologists has now expanded to include intensivists, emergency physicians, and a wide range of healthcare professionals. The increasing accessibility and portability of ultrasound technology have made it an indispensable tool for bedside diagnosis and management.

PULSE: Emergency Ultrasound Guide is specifically designed for frontline physicians, residents, and medical students who are looking for a practical and concise guide to emergency ultrasound. Whether you work in emergency departments, general wards, intensive care units (ICUs), or other acute care settings, this book aims to provide you with the essential knowledge and skills to integrate ultrasound into your daily practice.

This comprehensive guide covers the use of ultrasound to rapidly diagnose a wide range of conditions, from head to toe. The book is organized into logical sections, each focusing on a specific area of the body. The content is intentionally concise, with a focus on practical aspects and omitting unnecessary details.

Throughout the book, you will find numerous images, diagrams, and illustrations that enhance understanding and provide a clear visual representation of ultrasound findings. The book also includes practical tips, pearls, and pitfalls to help you navigate the complexities of emergency ultrasound.

This book is specifically designed with the novice in mind, aiming to empower them with the fundamentals of ultrasonography and inspire its integration into their daily practice. Ultimately, we envision that physicians of all levels will benefit from the content, enhancing their clinical decision-making and improving patient outcomes.

Editorial Team

Acknowledgments

We acknowledge with gratitude the contributions of our team members who made this handbook possible. Special appreciation goes to our esteemed authors, whose outstanding dedication and expertise played a pivotal role in shaping the content of this book.

We are deeply indebted to the patients who generously allowed us to publish their scans, enabling us to enhance educational value and advance medical knowledge.

We extend our heartfelt appreciation to the team of M/s Jaypee Brothers Medical Publishers (P) Ltd, New Delhi, India, for their unwavering dedication, tireless efforts, and unrelenting commitment to excellence.

We express our sincere gratitude to our colleagues and families, whose daily encouragement and unwavering support were instrumental in our success.

Editorial Team

A very special acknowledgement goes to my son Pravi Maitreya and my parents, whose constant support, love, and inspiration have been my greatest strength throughout this journey.

Alka Verma

Contents

CHAPTER 1

Knobology and Image Optimization

Harshit Agarwal, Vijeta Bajpai

WHAT YOU WILL LEARN IN THIS CHAPTER?

A. Components of an ultrasound (US) machine
B. Use of different transducers
C. Use of various buttons in US machine
D. Image optimization

INTRODUCTION

Knobology encompasses the study of the various controls and adjustments that are used to optimize imaging. Understanding the knobology of ultrasonography (USG) is essential for both novice and experienced practitioners to ensure accurate diagnoses and effective use for patient care.[1]

BASIC PRINCIPLE OF ULTRASOUND

Ultrasonography operates on a straightforward principle: a transducer emits sound waves that bounce off tissues, and returning echoes are received and converted into images. Viewed in real-time on a monitor, these images allow healthcare providers to assess organs, blood flow, and various bodily structures. The effectiveness of this imaging technique largely depends on the operator's ability to manipulate the controls of the ultrasound machine—hence the importance of learning knobology.

COMPONENTS OF AN ULTRASOUND MACHINE

Before diving into the specifics of knobology, it is essential to understand the primary components of an ultrasound machine:

- *Transducer:* The device that emits and receives sound waves. Different transducers are used for various applications, such as abdominal, obstetric, or cardiac imaging.
- *Control panel:* This is where the knobology comes into play. The control panel houses various knobs, buttons, and touchscreen interfaces that allow the operator to manipulate the ultrasound settings **(Fig. 1)**.
- *Monitor:* Displays real-time images generated by the transducer, allowing the operator to assess the quality and clarity of the images.

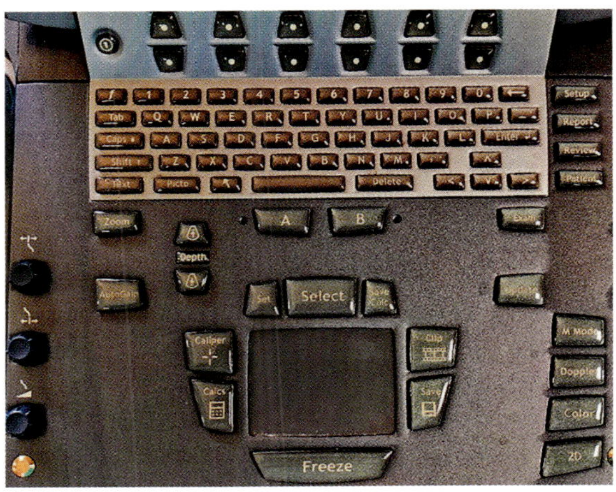

Fig. 1: Keyboard of an ultrasound (USG) machine.

- *Printer:* Some ultrasound machines are equipped with printers to produce hard copies of images for patient records.

TRANSDUCERS

An ultrasound transducer converts electrical energy into mechanical (sound) energy and back again, based on the piezoelectric effect.

- It is the handheld part of the ultrasound machine that is responsible for the production and detection of ultrasound waves.
- Different types of transducers exist. However, three main types of transducers used for emergency sonography are (A) Linear; (B) Curvilinear; and (C) Cardiac (phased array) probe **(Figs. 2A to C)**.
- The choice of probe depends upon the organ to be scanned and depth of the tissue.[2]
- Curvilinear probes have a lower frequency and a wider footprint and are hence useful for imaging deeper structures such as intra-abdominal organs or lungs.
- The cardiac phased array probe has a smaller footprint, which aids in imaging between the ribs. It generates ultrasound from an electronically steered beam in a close array, providing high penetration depth and high temporal resolution (i.e., frame rate). Consequently, the echo probe can accurately display the entire heart, including moving structures such as valves.

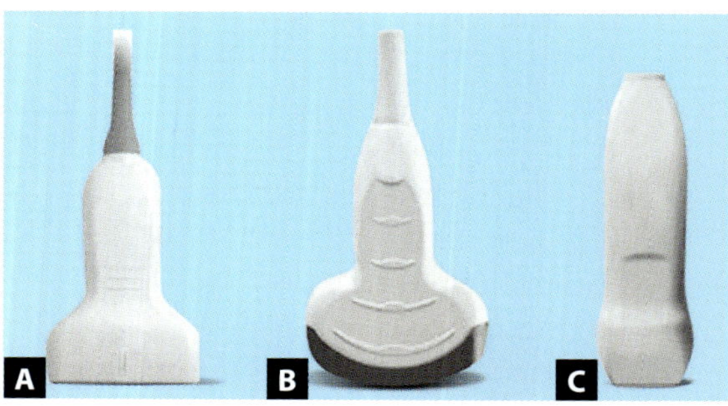

Figs. 2A to C: Different types of transducers. (A) Linear probe; (B) Curvilinear probe; (C) Cardiac (phased array) probe.

- Linear/vascular probes have high frequency, better for imaging superficial blood vessels, and tissues like the thyroid, breast, musculoskeletal tissue, etc.
- Both curvilinear and phased array probes generate "pie-shaped" images on the screen, which are narrower in the near field and wider in the distant field. In contrast, linear probes produce rectangular images on the screen. Thus, by observing the monitor and the images obtained, it is possible to determine which probe was used for scanning.

IMPORTANT KNOBS IN CLINICAL USE

- *Power/on-off button:*
  - This is usually situated on the top left corner of the machine but the position differs from manufacturer to manufacturer. What does not differ is the universal symbol of power/on-off button.
  - If the ultrasound machine does not turn on after pressing the power button, check if the power cord is plugged in properly in the machine. The power cord should be snuggly fit in the socket and should not wobble.
  - If the power cord is properly fitted and the machine is not still switching on, check if the electricity switch is turned on following which try switching on the machine by plugging the cord in a different socket.
- *Gain selector* ***(Figs. 3A to C)****:*
  - Ultrasound waves traveling through various tissue planes reduce in strength due to absorption and up to a small extent dispersal. Once the waves are reflected back toward the transducer, the attenuation in the signal continues due to the above-mentioned phenomena

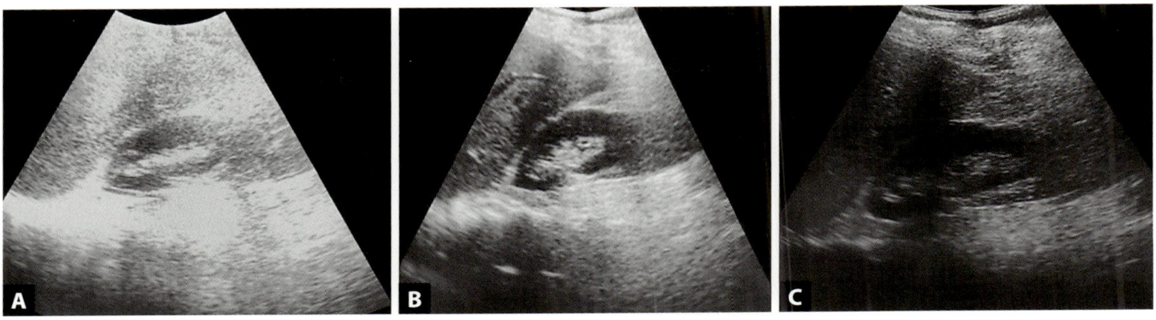

Figs. 3A to C: Impact of gain on visibility. (A) Too high; (B) Appropriate; (C) Too low.

reducing echoes from deep structures. Therefore, the structure under evaluation will seem hyperechoic on bringing it closer to the transducer or hypoechoic if moved away from the transducer.

- The gain function of the ultrasound machine mitigates the attenuation of USG signal strength. Gain works by increasing/decreasing the amplification of the signal strength returning to the transducer.
- The manipulation of the gain function appears as the brightening or dimming of the image displayed on the monitor, much like what we observe on domestic television sets and computer monitors. Higher gain increases the brightness (apparent echogenicity) of the image **(Fig. 3A)** while lowering the gain darkens it **(Fig. 3C)**. Initially, overusing or underusing the gain button after acquiring the image can help to understand the function and fine-tune of the acquired image for diagnostic decisions and procedures.
- An appropriately adjusted image **(Fig. 3B)** will show fluid (anechoic structure) as black and solid tissues will appear along the spectrum of gray to white (hypoechoic, isoechoic, and hyperechoic). Defining an image as hyperechoic, isoechoic, or hypoechoic is usually based on using liver as a reference range. Traditionally, a scan of the liver with gallbladder is used as a reference. The liver must appear gray (isoechoic). Gallbladder without sludge gives black image (anechoic).[3]

- *Depth setter* ***(Figs. 4A and B)****:*
  - The depth of the image needs to be adjusted to acquire and position the structure under evaluation to the center of the monitor.
  - Start scanning with a greater "depth" than required so as to visualize the surrounding structures too. Doing so is strongly advised while doing ultrasound-guided procedures as it helps in building a better spatial orientation for the person doing the procedure and aids in better accuracy. Once the image of the target structure is acquired, the depth of the image should be adjusted to place the area of interest in the center of the screen.
  - If the depth is set shallow **(Fig. 4A)**/deeper **(Fig. 4B)** than appropriate, the target structure has poor resolution and some informations may be missed in such scans. A major limiting factor with compact portable ultrasound machines commonly used in emergency departments and ICUs is that these devices have a fixed zone of focus. Hence the operator must adjust the depth function to focus the target structure to the monitor's center.

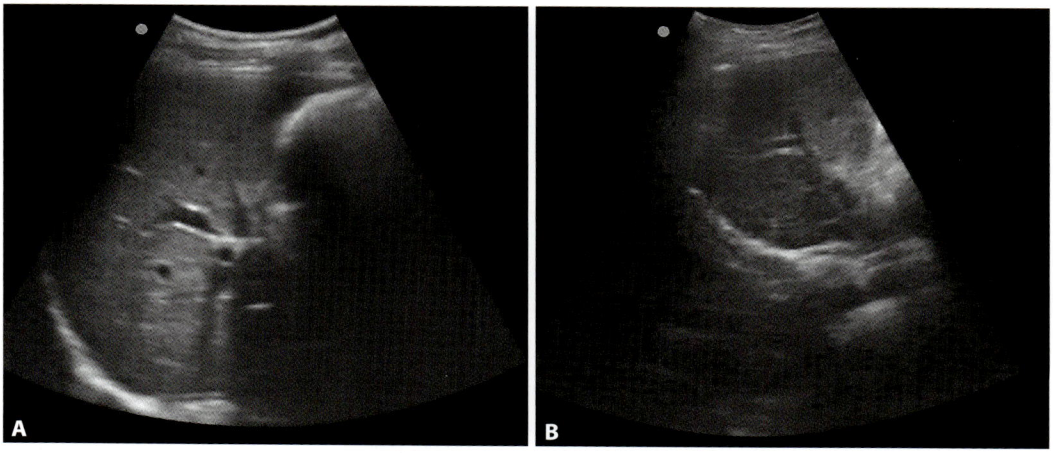

Figs. 4A and B: Impact of depth on visibility. (A) Too shallow; (B) Too deep.

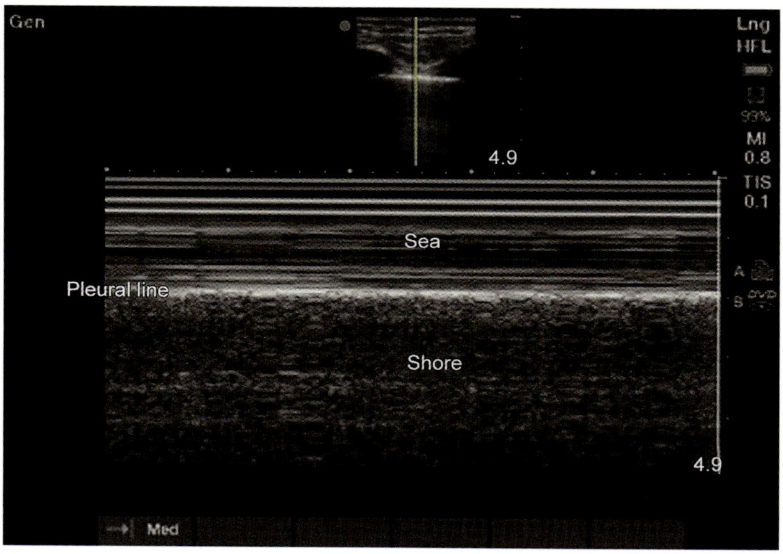

Fig. 5: Pleural sliding along the green line.

- *Mode selector:* Ultrasound machines have multiple imaging modalities.
  - *Brightness mode/B-mode*: It is a default mode of USG that produces two-dimensional gray images.
  - *Motion mode/M-mode* ***(Fig. 5)****:* It displays motion of structures over time and is particularly useful in cardiac ultrasound and visualizing pleural sliding sign during lung ultrasound. The motion mode shows the movement of the entire structure over time along the single scan line. Due to the high frame/sampling rate of M-mode, it gives a good resolution of rapidly moving structures.

The scan is begun by centering the target structure on the screen. The "M-mode" scanning line (green line) is then directed

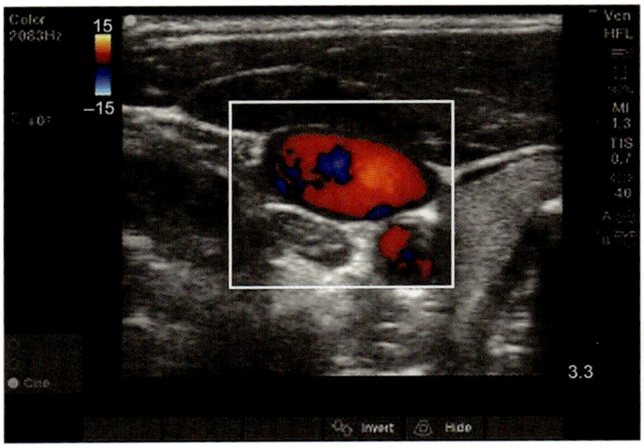

Fig. 6: Color Doppler mode on ultrasonography (USG).

across the area of interest. The “M-mode” button is then pressed again to display the movement of the structure over a certain time.

- *Color Doppler mode* ***(Fig. 6)****:* It displays blood flow based on its direction relative to probe. Blood flowing away from the probe appears blue while toward it appears red. Color of flow on the monitor does not signify its venous or arterial nature or its oxygenation status. The color map on the screen displays the corresponding Doppler shift. The gain for color Doppler mode is adjusted in a similar manner as the gain of B-mode. Once color Doppler mode is activated, gain is adjusted in a manner that some pixels are visible on the screen intermittently with most of the color box black.[4]

- *Freeze/image capture:* The freeze button screenshots the live image being displayed and freezes the screen. Once the image is frozen/captured, it can be printed (for documentation) or used for measurements, e.g., inferior vena cava diameter, a static parameter to assess the fluid status of the patient.
- *Caliper and measuring button* ***(Figs. 7A and B)****:* Once an image is acquired and the target structure properly focused, these buttons will produce cursors on the screen to measure the distances.

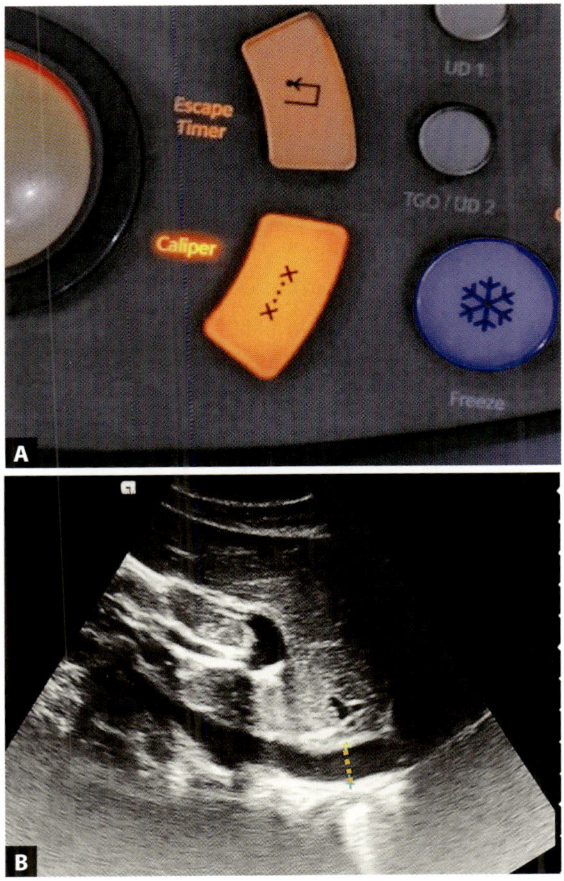

Figs. 7A and B: Caliper button and measurement.

IMAGE OPTIMIZATION

Mastering the knobology of USG is not merely about understanding the controls; it is about knowing when and how to adjust them to optimize the image quality. Several factors influence the effectiveness of ultrasound imaging, including patient characteristics, the area of interest, and the specific clinical question being addressed.

- *Patient factors:* Body habitus, age, and specific medical conditions can all impact ultrasound imaging. For instance, a patient with a larger body habitus may require adjustments in gain and depth to achieve optimal imaging.
- *Clinical context:* Different clinical scenarios necessitate different imaging techniques. For example, obstetric ultrasounds require different settings than abdominal or cardiac ultrasounds. Knowledge of these contexts helps operators make informed decisions regarding knob adjustments. In some newer machines, specific predetermined settings are available for specific regional or contextual imaging, e.g., echo preset, lungs preset, abdominal preset, and vascular preset. Using appropriate presets can also improve image quality.
- *Image interpretation:* An operator's ability to interpret images is directly linked to their proficiency with the machine's controls. By mastering knobology, practitioners can ensure that they capture the best possible images for accurate interpretation.[5]

CONCLUSION

Knobology is an integral aspect of USG. It is the knowledge and skill required to manipulate the controls of ultrasound machines effectively. Understanding the various knobs and their functions is crucial for optimizing image quality and ensuring accurate diagnoses. As the technology continues to advance, so will the complexity and capabilities of these machines, making proficiency in knobology more essential than ever. Through dedicated training, mentorship, and continuous education, practitioners can master this vital aspect of medical imaging, ultimately enhancing patient care and outcomes.

REFERENCES

1. Enriquez JL, Wu TS. An introduction to ultrasound equipment and knobology. Crit Care Clin. 2014;30(1):25-45, v.
2. Sehmbi H, Perlas A. Basics of ultrasound imaging. In: Jankovic D, Peng P (Eds). Regional Nerve Blocks in Anesthesia and Pain Therapy: Imaging-guided and Traditional Techniques. Cham: Springer International Publishing; 2022. pp. 33-52.
3. MacDonald D. Basics of ultrasound. In: MacDonald D (Ed). Oral and Maxillofacial Radiology: A Diagnostic Approach. USA: Wiley-Blackwell; 2019. pp. 151-8.
4. Chassot PG. Basic principles of Doppler ultrasound. In: Transesophageal Echocardiography Multimedia Manual, 1st edition. Boca Raton: CRC Press; 2005. pp. 51-68.
5. Wu Q, Li X, Li L, Yan O, He Q. Analysis of factors affecting ultrasound examination time: A quantitative study. Technol Health Care. 2023;32(2):1015-27.

CHAPTER 2

Neuro Ultrasound

Nidhi Singh, Suruchi Ambasta

WHAT YOU WILL LEARN IN THIS CHAPTER?

A. Basic anatomy and physiology of optic nerve sheath diameter (ONSD)

B. Clinical application of ONSD in emergency department

INTRODUCTION

The eye reflects the acoustic properties of the brain under pressure and offers a unique perspective on neurological health. Use of ultrasound for measurement of optic nerve sheath diameter (ONSD) is a straightforward and reliable method for assessment of intracranial pressure (ICP). ONSD measurements serve as a vital diagnostic tool, bridging the eye's anatomy with the underlying dynamics of brain function.

WHY OPTIC NERVE SHEATH DIAMETER?

The eye is appropriate for imaging via ultrasound because of its superficial location with distinct, fluid-filled structures that provide a perfect medium for transmitting ultrasound beams. The optic nerve emerges from the posterior orbit and is encircled by a meningeal layer known as the optic nerve sheath. The sheath contains a small and circumferential compartment of cerebrospinal fluid which is in continuation with the intracranial subarachnoid space.[1] Accordingly, any change in the ICP is mirrored in the diameter of the optic nerve sheath. As an extension of the brain, the optic nerve responds to changes in ICP. An increased pressure causes an expansion of the subarachnoid space and, consequently, the optic nerve sheath. Monitoring of ONSD provides a valuable, practical means of assessing changes in ICP.[1,2]

OPTIC NERVE SHEATH DIAMETER AND INTRACRANIAL PRESSURE

Elevated ICP is a life-threatening situation ensuing from multiple pathological conditions, such as cerebral edema, intracranial hemorrhage, subarachnoid hemorrhage, and brain tumors. The use of invasive ICP-monitoring devices, like intraventricular catheters, is the gold standard for monitoring ICP. However, there are chances of misplacement, infection, hemorrhage, and obstruction. Additionally, intraparenchymal catheters and pneumatic sensors may not always be available. Shifting patients to neuroimaging may be risky.

Assessment of ONSD through the ocular window is a safe alternative due to low cost, rapid bedside application, and lack of radiation exposure.[2] Early detection via ultrasound allows for prompt therapeutic action, potentially improving patient outcomes in patients with intracranial hypertension.

Optic nerve sheath diameter is primarily used as a screening tool for increased ICP. The cutoff value of ONSD indicating raised ICP remains ambiguous in the literature. No single cutoff value has been established as a definitive indicator for urgent intervention. A threshold of 0.5 cm (5 mm) is commonly used to screen for raised ICP. A 2023 systemic review and meta-analysis suggested a cutoff range of 5.6–6.3 mm to be highly specific for diagnosing elevated ICP, without significantly compromising sensitivity.[3]

TECHNIQUE OF MEASURING OPTIC NERVE SHEATH DIAMETER[4]

Preparation

- *Ultrasound machine preparation:*
  - *Transducer:* Select a high-frequency linear probe (7–10 MHz). Set the ultrasound machine to visualize structures up to 5–6 cm deep.
  - *Ultrasound machine placement:* Position the ultrasound machine on the patient's right side, enabling you to scan with your right hand while adjusting the machine's controls with your left hand **(Figs. 1A and B)**.
- *Patient preparation:*
  - The patient should be fully supine, though the head of the bed can be elevated up to 45° if needed.
  - Apply ultrasound gel generously to the closed eye ensuring that the ultrasound probe does not exert excessive pressure on the patient's eye. A Tegaderm patch is preferably placed over the closed eye of interest.
  - Rest the hand bearing the probe on the forehead of the patient or place your little finger on the nose of patient or the zygomatic arch to avoid direct pressure on the globe and ensure patient's comfort **(Figs. 2A and B)**.

Identifying the Optic Nerve Sheath

- *Probe positioning:* Adjust the probe by making small side-to-side movements and gently angle it either superiorly or inferiorly to show the ingress of the anechoic optic nerve into the globe **(Fig. 3)**.
- *Image capture:* After obtaining the best possible view, the image is saved as a single frame or as a video loop and the probe is removed from the eye.
- *Patient instruction:* If the patient is awake, instruct them to keep their eyes closed and

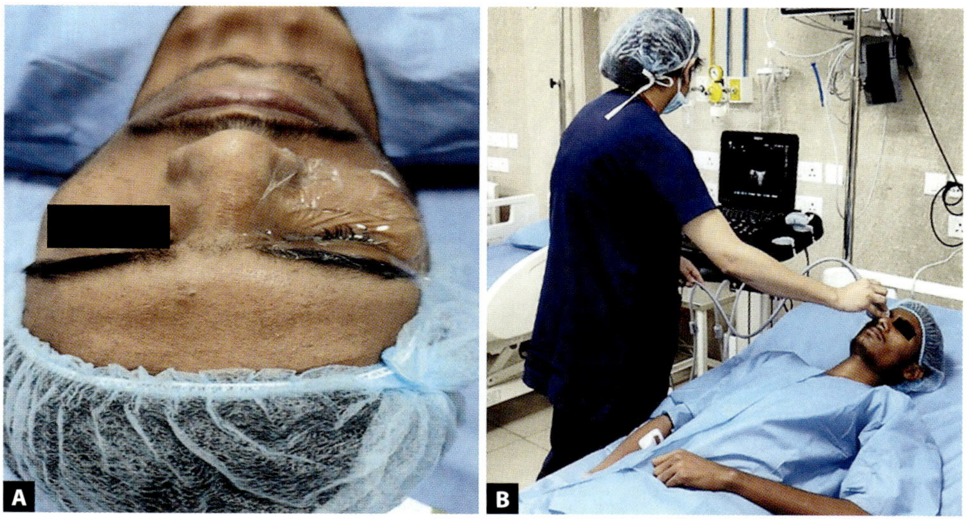

Figs. 1A and B: *Preparation:* Patient and machine positioning.

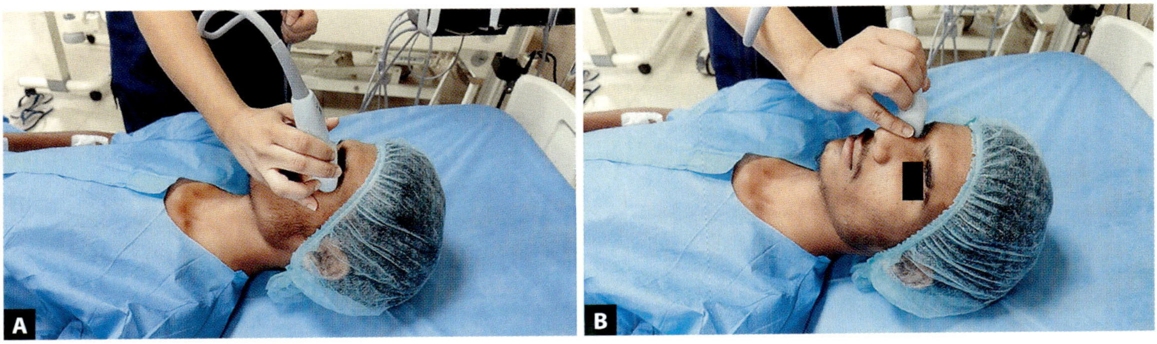

Figs. 2A and B: *Probe placement on bony prominences:* (A) Left eye—anchor on zygomatic arch; (B) Right eye—anchor on nose.

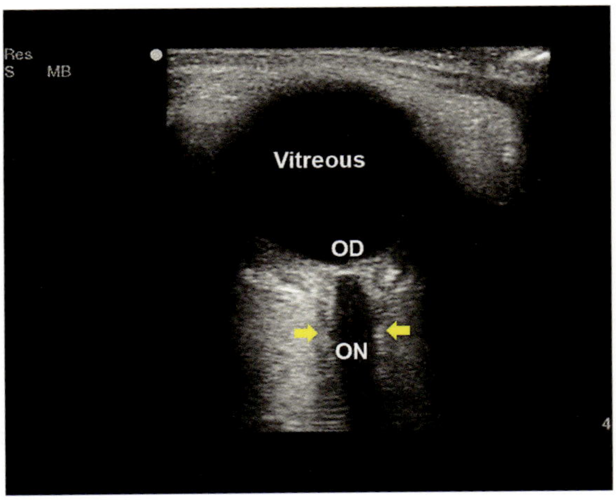

Fig. 3: Identification of optic nerve and optic nerve sheath. (OD: optic disk; ON: optic nerve; Yellow horizontal arrows: optic nerve sheath)

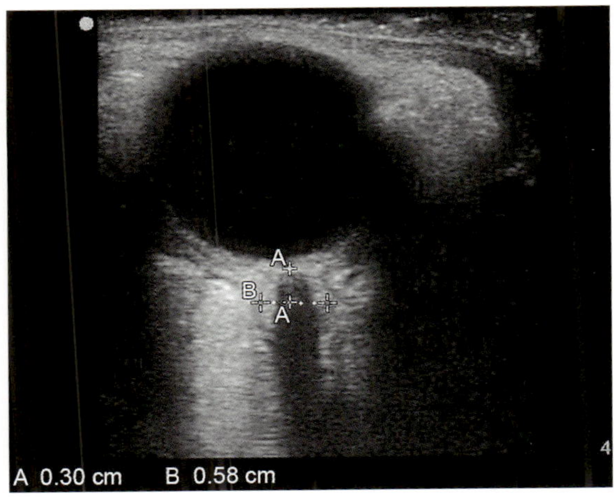

Fig. 4: Measurement of optic nerve sheath diameter (ONSD) (the ONSD is measured 3 mm behind the retina where a transverse line is drawn to measure the outer edge of optic sheath).

look straight ahead during the procedure to ensure accurate imaging.

Measuring Optic Nerve Sheath Diameter

- Use the "caliper" function of the ultrasound machine to measure precisely.
- Draw a 3-mm vertical reference line from the juncture of the optic nerve and the eyeball. At this point, draw a horizontal line across the optic nerve to get the diameter of the optic nerve sheath in millimeters **(Fig. 4)**.
- To ensure accuracy, average two or three measurements taken from each side

PEARLS AND PITFALLS

Overall advantages and disadvantages of ONSD have been outlined in **Table 1**. Various practical pearls and pitfalls regarding ONSD are discussed here.

Potential False Positives

Following conditions can lead to increased ONSD without a corresponding elevation in ICP:

TABLE 1: Advantages and disadvantages of ONSD.

Advantages	*Disadvantages*
• Noninvasive technique • Can be measured rapidly at the patient's bedside • Safe, does not involve any ionizing radiation exposure • Cost-effective when compared to other imaging modalities • Useful in resource-limited settings • Portable equipment and patient transportation are not required • Repeatable, allows frequent monitoring of ICP trends over time • Good intra and interobserver reproducibility	• Lack of uniform cutoff • Operator dependant • Risk of pressure injury to the globe • Severe coagulopathies and globe rupture are the contraindications to performing ONSD measurements • Movement of the eyeball, preexisting structural anomalies of eye and anatomical lesions may influence the ONSD

(ICP: intracranial pressure; ONSD: optic nerve sheath diameter)

- Optic neuritis
- Optic nerve glioma or meningioma
- Inflammatory infiltration
- Cavernous sinus masses
- Graves' orbitopathy
- Leukemic infiltration
- Orbital congestion with sheath swelling.

Hence, underlying medical and neurological conditions must be considered while interpreting ONSD values. In a few patients, a thorough evaluation by a neurologist and/or an ophthalmologist may be necessary to differentiate between elevated ICP and other causes of ONSD enlargement.

Where to Measure?

- It is to be remembered that anatomically optic nerve sheath is a complex system (including arachnoid trabeculae, pillars, and septa which compartmentalize the subarachnoid space) and not a perfectly circular structure. Hence, a standard reference point is needed for measuring ONSD.
- The ONSD is typically measured at the point where the optic nerve enters the eyeball, i.e., 3 mm posterior to the vitreoretinal junction. This point is also believed to be the site where maximum changes due to raised ICP can be observed, along the long axis of the optic nerve.
- Here, the horizontal measurement should be taken from the outer edges of the nerve sheath, not the inner edges of the optic nerve itself.[2,4] This is because the expansion of the optic nerve sheath reflects the fluctuations in ICP which the measurement of optic nerve diameter alone fails to do.
- Obtain both horizontal and vertical measurements for each eye to enhance the accuracy of the ONSD assessment **(Figs. 5A and B)**.

Optic Nerve Sheath Diameter Cutoff

The optimal cutoff values for ONSD as an indicator of elevated ICP are not clearly defined, with studies suggesting a range from 4.9 to 6.3 mm.[4,5] Although a cutoff of around 5.0 mm is commonly used, variability in patient demographics, clinical settings, and measurement techniques complicates the establishment of a definitive standard. The sensitivity and specificity for detecting ICP ≥20 mm Hg range from 74 to 100% and 63 to 95%, respectively, depending on the specific cutoff used.[5] Meta-analyses struggle to produce pooled sensitivity and specificity due to this variability, highlighting the need to interpret ONSD in the context of the overall clinical picture rather than as a standalone diagnostic tool. Rather than relying on a single absolute value, it is important to observe trends in ONSD measurements.[3,5]

Safety

To ensure the safety of the optic globe and prevent damage to sensitive structures such as the retina

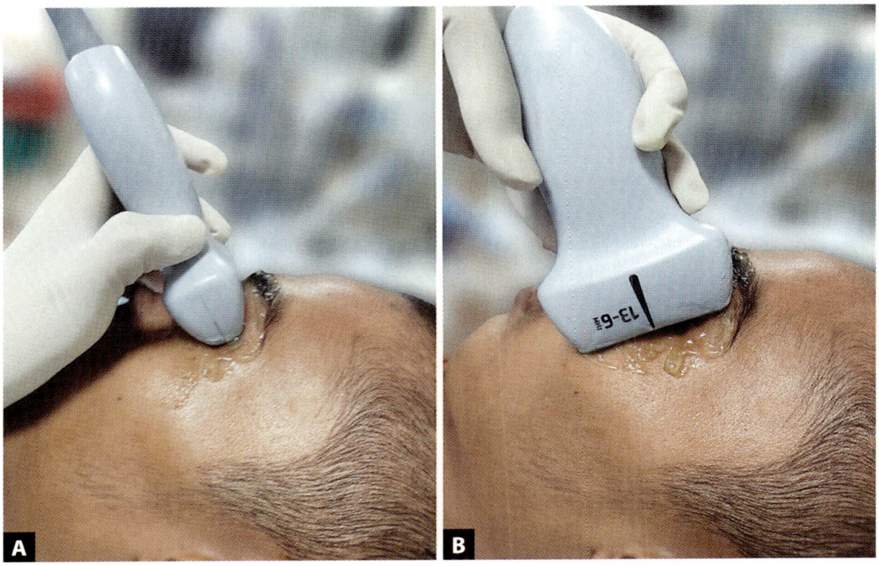

Figs. 5A and B: *Lateral views of probe position:* (A) Horizontal; (B) Vertical probe placement.

and lens, the Food and Drug Administration (FDA) has set specific maximum exposure limits for ophthalmic ultrasound. For ONSD measurements using ultrasound, it is crucial to follow the As Low As Reasonably Achievable (ALARA) principles to minimize potential biohazards. This includes reducing scan times, limiting acoustic power, and ensuring the mechanical index (MI) remains ≤0.23 and the thermal index (TI) ≤1.[6,7]

Also, scanning through the lens should be avoided to prevent potential thermal damage to it. Upon obtaining an optimal image, it is advisable to make measurements from stored frames or video loops to minimize active scanning time, thereby reducing unnecessary exposure to ultrasound energy.

Use Color Doppler

Using color Doppler to identify the ophthalmic artery, which runs along the optic nerve, enhances the accurate identification of the ONSD margins. The ophthalmic artery, along with the central retinal artery and central retinal vein, can be visualized during ONSD measurements. Identifying these vessels through Doppler imaging not only confirms the anatomical location of the optic nerve but also helps in precisely delineating the ONSD margins, ensuring accurate measurement and avoiding errors from surrounding structures or artifacts.[7]

CONCLUSION

Optic nerve sheath diameter measurement in emergency care is a valuable, noninvasive method for assessing elevated ICP when interpreted in conjunction with the patient's clinical presentation. This point-of-care ultrasound technique offers several advantages, including accessibility, cost-effectiveness, and minimal patient discomfort, making it highly suitable for resource-limited environments. The use of serial ONSD measurements allows clinicians to monitor ICP trends over time. However, proper training and adherence to standardized measurement protocols are required before initiating its use on patients.[7] High-frequency probes, color Doppler for vascular identification, and minimizing ultrasound exposure are essential elements of safe ONSD practice.

As research refines cutoff values for detecting raised ICP, emergency physicians need to stay current with best practices and emerging evidence. This ensures the optimal use of ONSD measurements, enhancing diagnostic accuracy and improving patient outcomes.

REFERENCES

1. De La Hoz Polo M, Torramilans Lluís A, Pozuelo Segura O, Anguera Bosque A, Esmerado Appiani C, Caminal Mitjana JM. Ocular ultrasonography focused on the posterior eye segment: what radiologists should know. Insights Imaging. 2016;7(3):351-64.
2. Shirodkar CG, Rao SM, Mutkule DP, Harde YR, Venkategowda PM, Mahesh MU. Optic nerve sheath diameter as a marker for evaluation and prognostication of intracranial pressure in Indian patients: an observational study. Indian J Crit Care Med. 2014;18(11):728-34.
3. Berhanu D, Ferreira JC, Abegão Pinto L, Aguiar de Sousa D, Lucas Neto L, Tavares Ferreira J. The role of optic nerve sheath ultrasonography in increased intracranial pressure: a systematic review and meta analysis. J Neurol Sci. 2023;454:120853.
4. Richards E, Munakomi S, Mathew D. Optic Nerve Sheath Ultrasound. In: StatPearls [Internet]. Treasure Island (FL): StatPearls Publishing; 2024.
5. Rajajee V, Vanaman M, Fletcher JJ, Jacobs TL. Optic nerve ultrasound for the detection of raised intracranial pressure. Neurocrit Care. 2011;15(3):506-15.
6. Lau T, Ahn JS, Manji R, Kim DJ. A Narrative review of point of care ultrasound assessment of the optic nerve in emergency medicine. Life (Basel). 2023;13(2):531.
7. Aspide R, Bertolini G, Albini Riccioli L, Mazzatenta D, Palandri G, Biasucci DG. A proposal for a new protocol for sonographic assessment of the optic nerve sheath diameter: the closed protocol. Neurocrit Care. 2020;32(1):327-32.

CHAPTER 3

Airway Ultrasound

Ruchi Verma

WHAT YOU WILL LEARN IN THIS CHAPTER?

A. Relevant anatomy of the upper airway

B. Sonoanatomy of airway

C. Applications of ultrasound in airway management

INTRODUCTION

Airway ultrasound is a simple, noninvasive, and bedside assessment of airway. Understanding the basic physics of ultrasound and being well-versed with upper airway anatomy are the keys to achieving expertise in performing it. Because of its shallow learning curve and ease of acquiring proficiency with training and availability of portable ultrasound machines in most of the critical areas, it is feasible to include it as part of airway management.

WHY AIRWAY ULTRASOUND IN EMERGENCY?

- Ultrasound enables us to identify different cartilages of the upper airway, cricothyroid membrane (CTM), and esophagus.
- Helps in identifying difficult mask ventilation and difficult intubation cases.
- Useful as a peri-intubation adjunct and assists in procedural guidance.
- Enhances first pass intubation success and ensures safety.

RELEVANT ANATOMY OF THE UPPER AIRWAY

- The anatomy of upper airway can be divided into suprahyoid and infrahyoid structures.
- Suprahyoid structures include mainly the tongue and below hyoid bone, thyrohyoid membrane, epiglottic, thyroid cartilage, vocal cords, CTM, cricoid cartilage, and tracheal rings are located craniocaudally.
- We can also view esophagus in suprasternal transverse view.
- Identification of all these structures in ultrasound is pivotal to the success of airway management **(Fig. 1)**.

ULTRASONIC CHARACTERISTICS OF DIFFERENT ELEMENTS OF AIRWAY

Air is a poor conductor of ultrasound waves, so it does not allow imaging of deeper structures of the airway. The presence of intraluminal air gives rise to both comet tail and reverberation artifacts. Various components of the airway appear divergently on ultrasonography **(Table 1)**.

STEPS OF AIRWAY ULTRASOUND

- *Patient position:*
    - Patients should be in a supine sniffing position with a pillow under the occiput for scanning suprahyoid structures. A neck extension is needed to scan infrahyoid structures.[1]

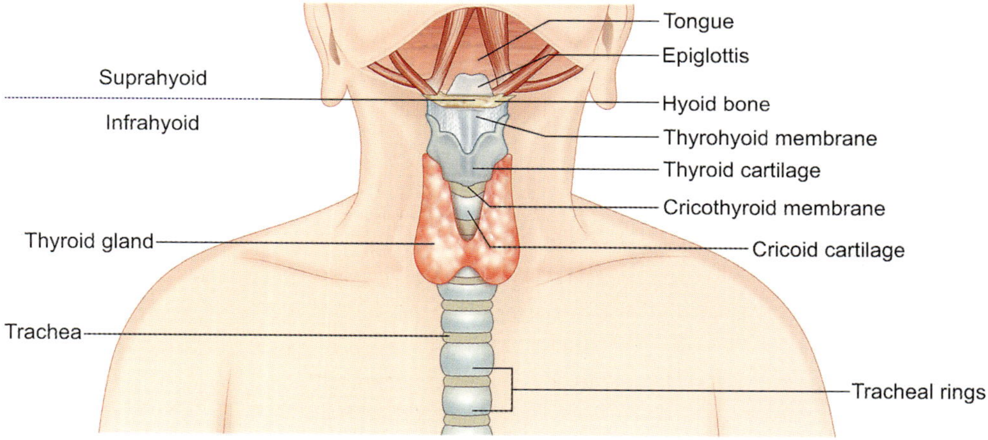

Fig. 1: Anatomy of upper airway.

TABLE 1: Ultrasonic characteristics of airway components.

Components	*Structures*	*Ultrasonic characteristic*
Cartilages	Epiglottis, thyroid cartilage, cricoid cartilage, and tracheal rings	Homogeneously hypoechoic (dark)
Bony structures	Hyoid bone and rami of the mandible/mentum	Hyperechoic (bright) linear structures with a hypoechoic acoustic shadow underneath
Air-mucosal interfaces	Anterior border of the air column	Hyperechoic (bright) line along the anterior border of the air column
Glandular structures	Thyroid gland	Homogeneous with medium echogenicity
Muscle and connective tissue	Strep muscles, tongue, thyrohyoid and cricothyroid membranes	Hypoechoic, heterogeneous striated appearance

- However, in trauma patients, we should rule out cervical spine injury before positioning the patient for the scan. In such scenarios, neck movement should be avoided, and the patient's neck should be kept in a neutral position to prevent cervical cord injury.

- *Probe selection and orientation:*
  - Linear and curvilinear ultrasound probes are most commonly used for visualizing the upper airway structures.
  - The probe is placed in the neck either in sagittal plane, parasagittal plane, or in the transverse plane.
  - A low frequency (3–8 MHz) curvilinear probe is used for scanning of deeper suprahyoid structures such as tongue base.
  - For hyoid and infrahyoid scanning, a high frequency (6–13 MHz) linear probe is more appropriate to visualize superficial structures such as epiglottis, thyroid cartilage, cricoid cartilage, and tracheal rings **(Figs. 2A and B)**.

Suprahyoid scan	Image acquisition	Noticeable structures
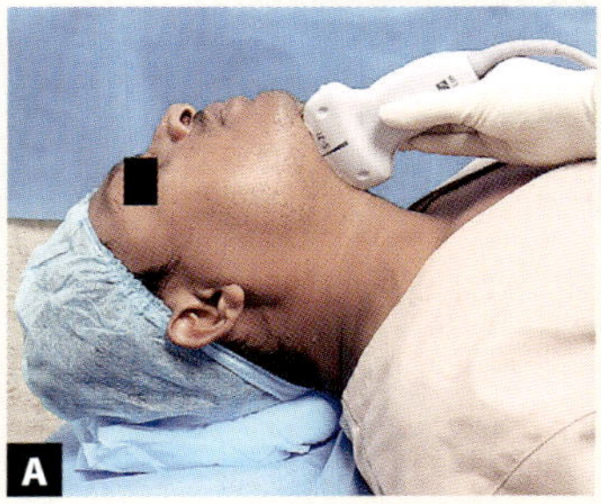	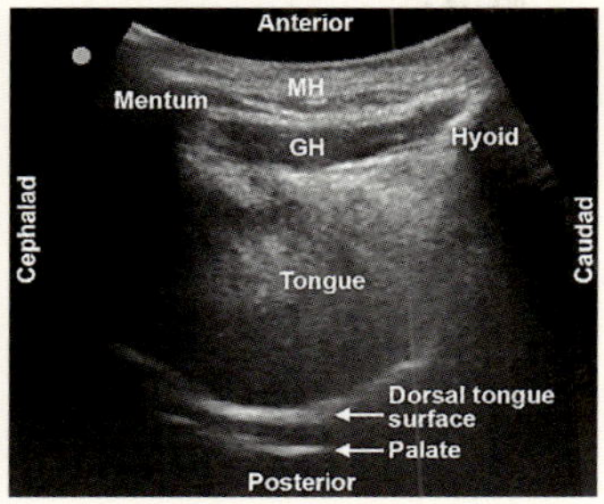	Base of the tongue and other oropharyngeal structures
Infrahyoid scan	**Image acquisition**	**Noticeable structures**
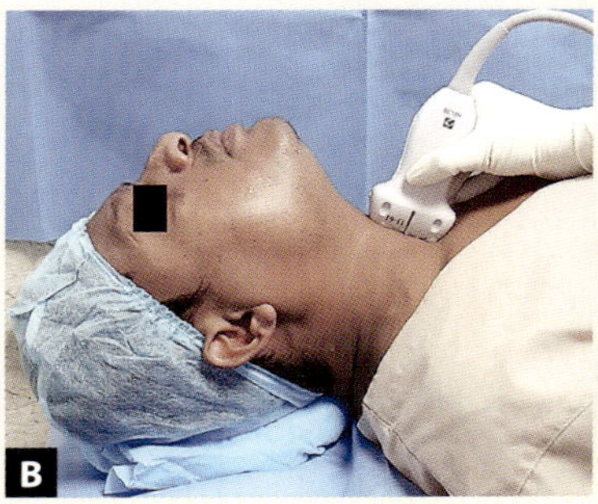	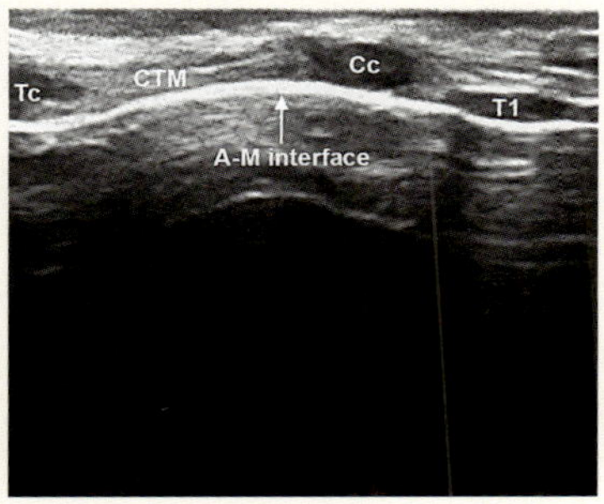	Epiglottis, thyroid cartilage (Tc), cricothyroid membrane (CTM), cricoid cartilage (Cc), tracheal ring (T1), and air-mucosa (A-M) interface

Figs. 2A and B: Ultrasound probe position for suprahyoid (A) and infrahyoid scan (B). (GH: geniohyoid muscles; MH: mylohyoid)

- *Sonoanatomy: Identification of structures on ultrasound*
  - Visualization of various structures of the airway on ultrasound utilizes different windows. Each ultrasound window is used for the identification of specific structures.[1]
  - The windows for obtaining images from above downward are suprahyoid, hyoid, thyrohyoid, thyroid, cricothyroid, cricoid, tracheal, and suprasternal **(Table 2)**.

APPLICATION/UTILITY OF ULTRASOUND IN AIRWAY MANAGEMENT

Ultrasound has a pertinent role in airway management. It is found useful in various ways during elective and emergency airway access.

- *Confirmation of endotracheal intubation:*
  - Obtaining an end-tidal CO_2 ($EtCO_2$) waveform is considered the gold standard method for confirmation of endotracheal intubation. $EtCO_2$ monitor may not be available in every hospital setting. Also, they are not reliable in low-perfusion states.
  - Ultrasound plays a vital role in such situations. It allows real-time visualization of endotracheal intubation and excludes esophageal intubation. In a study by Chaudhary et al., ultrasound was found to be a reliable and fastest method for confirming endotracheal intubation, compared to chest auscultation and capnography, with 100% sensitivity and specificity.[2]

TABLE 2: Ultrasonic windows for identification of airway structures.

Window	*Probe orientation*	*Structures identification*	*Sonographic appearance*
Suprahyoid	Sagittal	Tongue	Fan-shaped striated appearance with hyperechoic line on dorsal surface due to A-M interface **(Figs. 3A and B)**
Hyoid	Transverse	Hyoid bone	Hyperechoic inverted U-shaped linear structure with acoustic shadowing underneath **(Fig. 4)**
	Sagittal or parasagittal	Hyoid bone	Narrow curved structure with acoustic shadow artifact **(Fig. 5)**
Thyrohyoid	Transverse	Epiglottis	Hypoechoic curvilinear structure, with hyperechoic pre-epiglottic space (PES) and bright A-M interface depicting the posterior border **(Fig. 6)**
	Sagittal or parasagittal	Thyrohyoid membrane Epiglottis	Hyperechoic line between the hyoid bone and thyroid cartilage **(Fig. 5)** Hypoechoic longitudinal curvilinear structure
Thyroid	Transverse	Thyroid cartilage Vocal cords	"Inverted V-shaped" hypoechoic structure, with age-related hyperechogenic changes **(Fig. 7)** Isosceles triangle, deep to thyroid cartilage
	Sagittal or parasagittal	Thyroid cartilage	Hypoechoic linear structure **(Figs. 5 and 8)**
Cricothyroid	Sagittal	CTM	Longitudinal hyperechoic line connecting thyroid and cricoid cartilages with A-M interface posterior to it **(Fig. 8)**
	Transverse	CTM	Hyperechoic transverse line between the thyroid and cricoid cartilages with TACA technique
Cricoid	Sagittal	Cricoid cartilage	Largest oval hypoechoic structure like a "hump" **(Figs. 8 and 9)**
	Transverse	Cricoid cartilage	Hypoechoic "horseshoe-shaped" structure thicker than tracheal cartilage **(Fig. 10)**
Tracheal	Sagittal	Tracheal rings	Smaller hypoechoic oval structures, "string of pearl" appearance **(Fig. 9)**
	Transverse	Trachea	"Inverted U-shaped" hypoechoic structure with A-M interface posteriorly **(Fig. 11)**
Suprasternal	Transverse over suprasternal notch slightly toward left	Esophagus Trachea	Collapsed muscular structure with both hypo- and hyperechoic components, posterior-lateral toward the left of the trachea **(Fig. 12)**

(A-M: air-mucosal interface; CTM: cricothyroid membrane; TACA: thyroid-airline-cricoid-airline)

- Before attempting intubation, a linear ultrasound probe is placed just above the suprasternal notch in the transverse plane slightly toward the left.
- The esophagus can be identified as a collapsed muscular structure with both hypo- and hyperechoic components, usually located posterior-lateral slightly

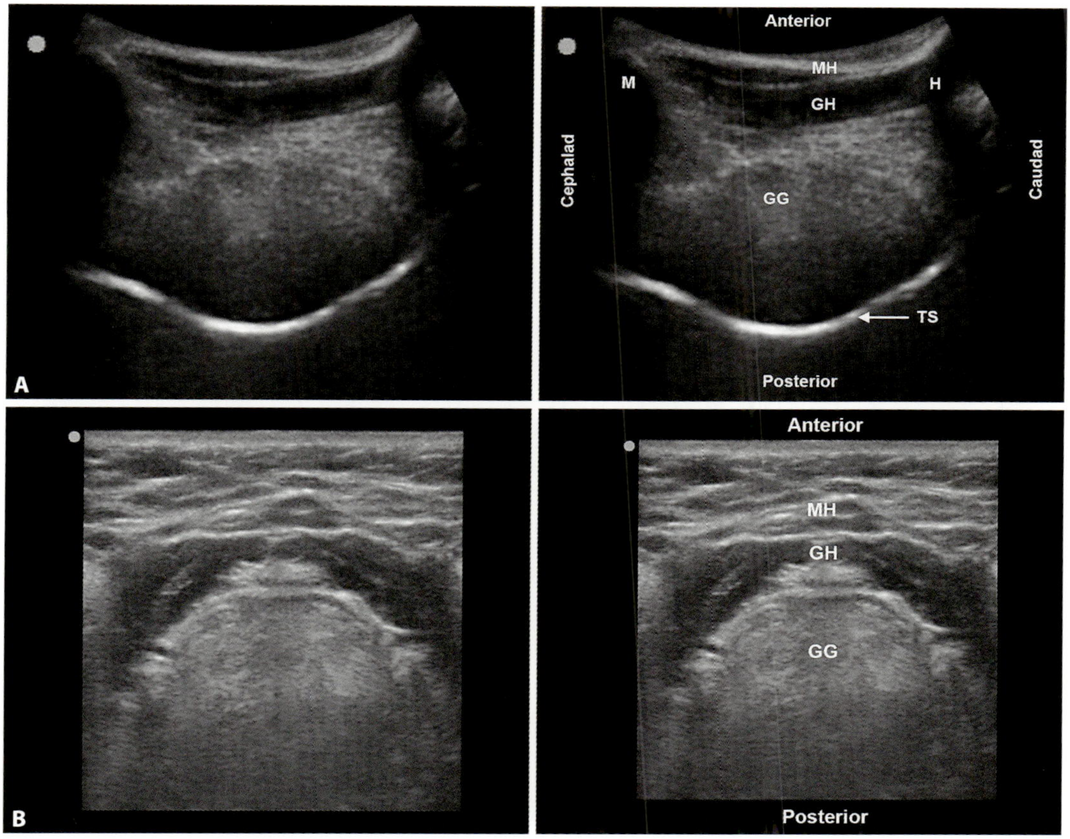

Figs. 3A and B: (A) Suprahyoid sagittal view; (B) Suprahyoid transverse view. (GG: genioglossus muscle; GH: geniohyoid muscle; MH: mylohyoid muscle, TS: dorsal tongue surface)

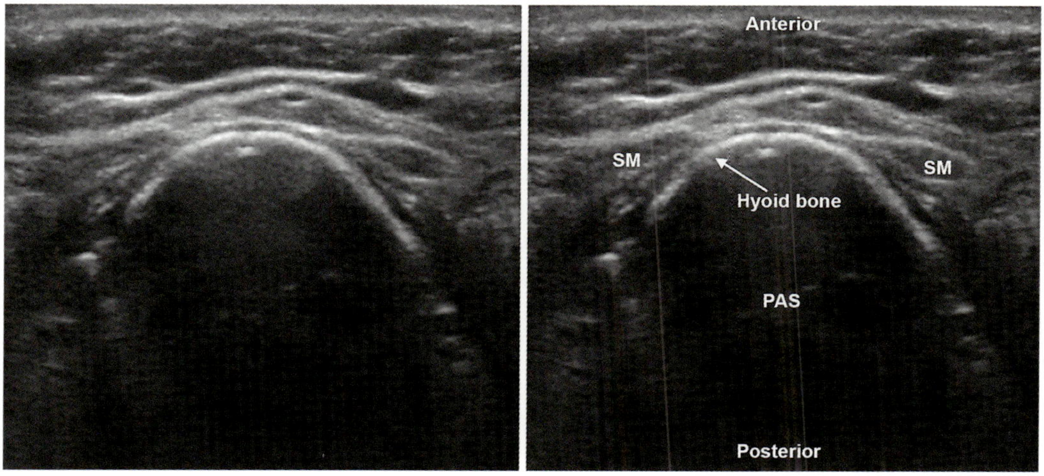

Fig. 4: Transverse view at hyoid bone level. (PA: posterior acoustic shadowing; SM: strap muscle)

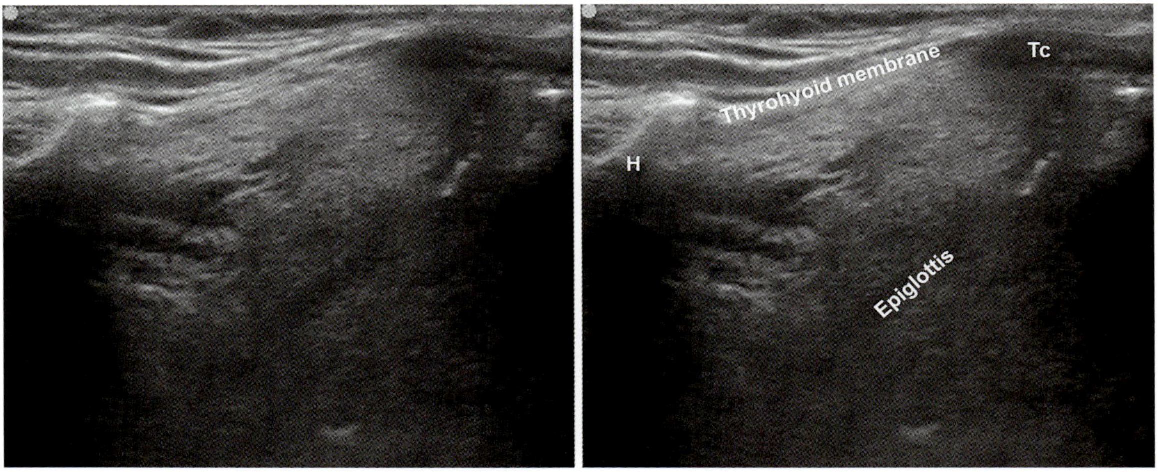

Fig. 5: Sagittal view through thyrohyoid membrane. (H: hyoid bone; Tc: thyroid cartilage)

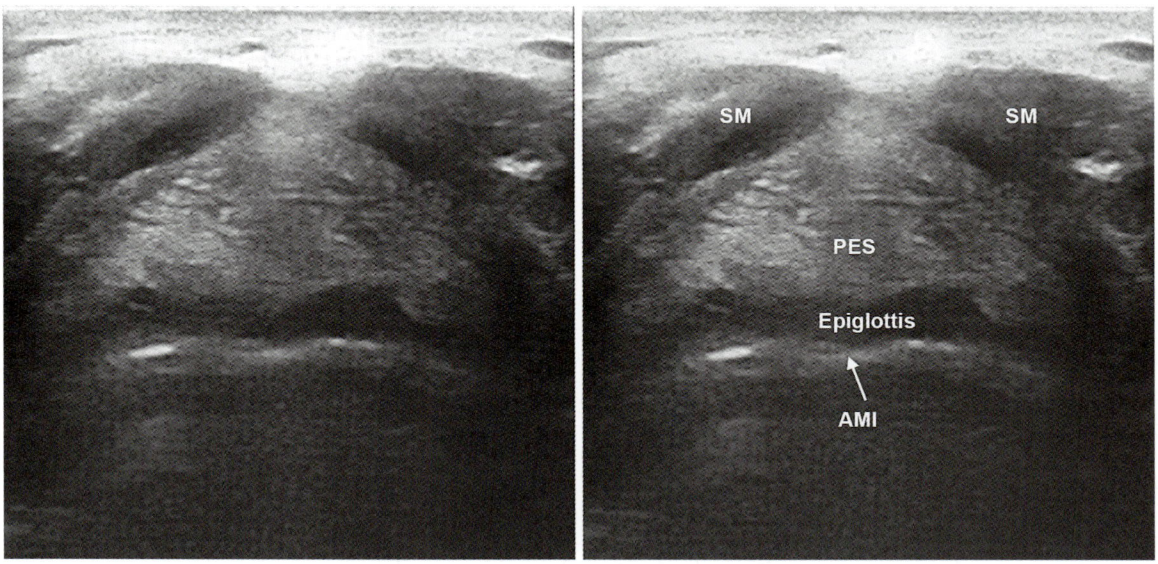

Fig. 6: Transverse view through thyrohyoid membrane showing epiglottis. (AMI: air-mucosal interface; PES: pre-epiglottic space; SM: strap muscle)

toward the left of the trachea. In an awake state, asking the patient for deglutition can help in identification.

- Tracheal intubation usually is a diagnosis of exclusion. In real-time ultrasonography, the dynamic opening of the esophageal lumen upon intubation in esophagus can be appreciated with the appearance of the second air-mucosal (A-M) interface with posterior artifacts on the described

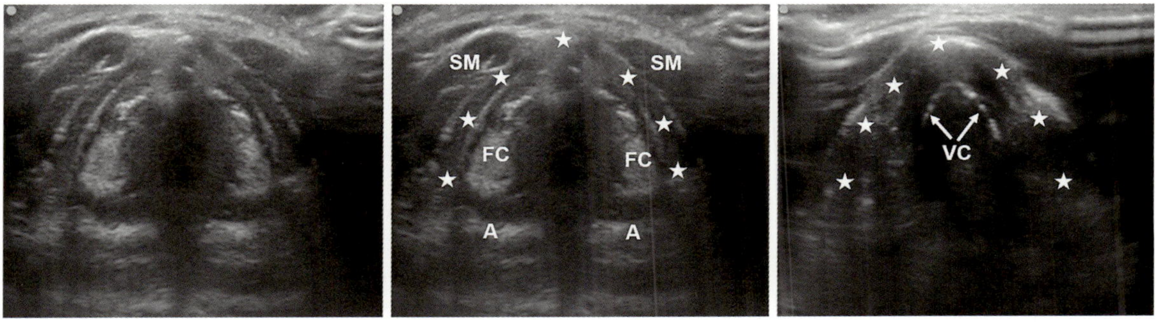

Fig. 7: Transverse view through thyroid cartilage. (A: arytenoid; FC: false cords; SM: strap muscle; VC: vocal cords; Stars: thyroid cartilage)

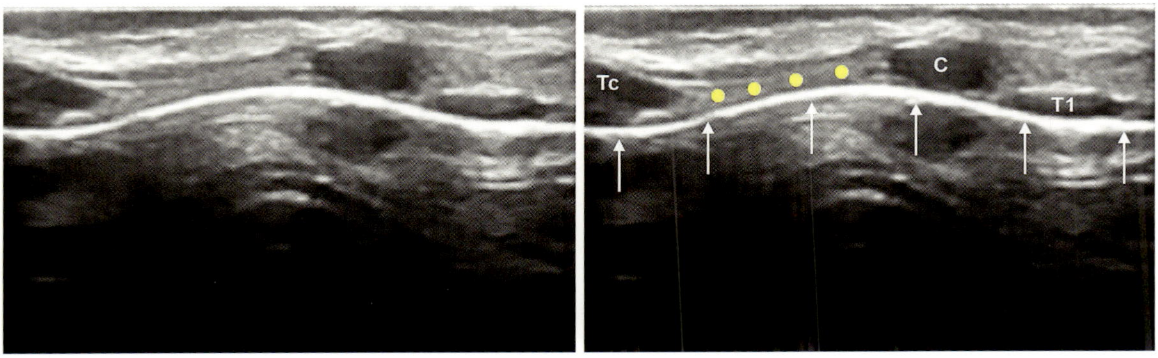

Fig. 8: Sagittal view showing cricothyroid membrane between thyroid and cricoid cartilages. (Arrow: air-mucosal interface; C: cricoid cartilage; Tc: thyroid cartilage; T1: first tracheal ring; Yellow dots: cricothyroid membrane)

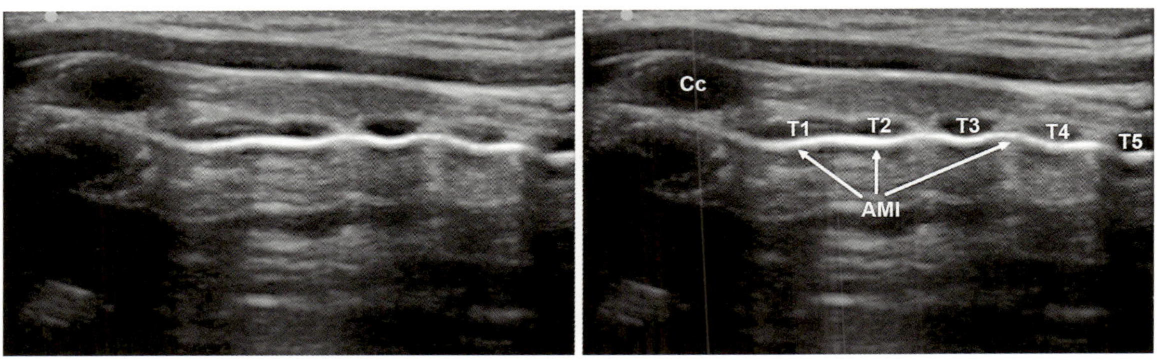

Fig. 9: Sagittal view over trachea showing tracheal rings as "string of pearls". (AMI: air-mucosal interface; Cc: cricoid cartilage; T1, T2, T3, T4, T5: tracheal rings)

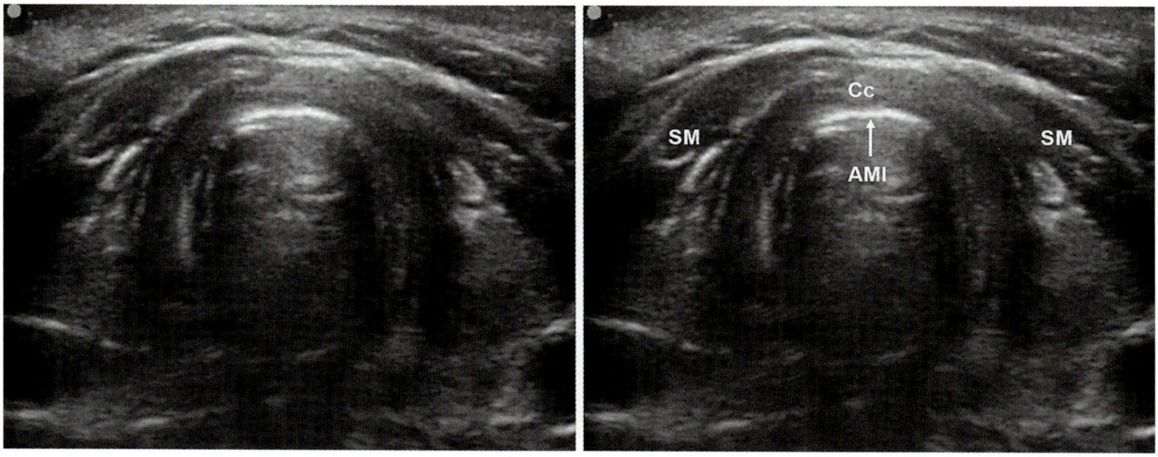

Fig. 10: Transverse view showing "horseshoe-shaped" cricoid cartilage. (AMI: air-mucosal interface; Cc: cricoid cartilage; SM: strap muscle)

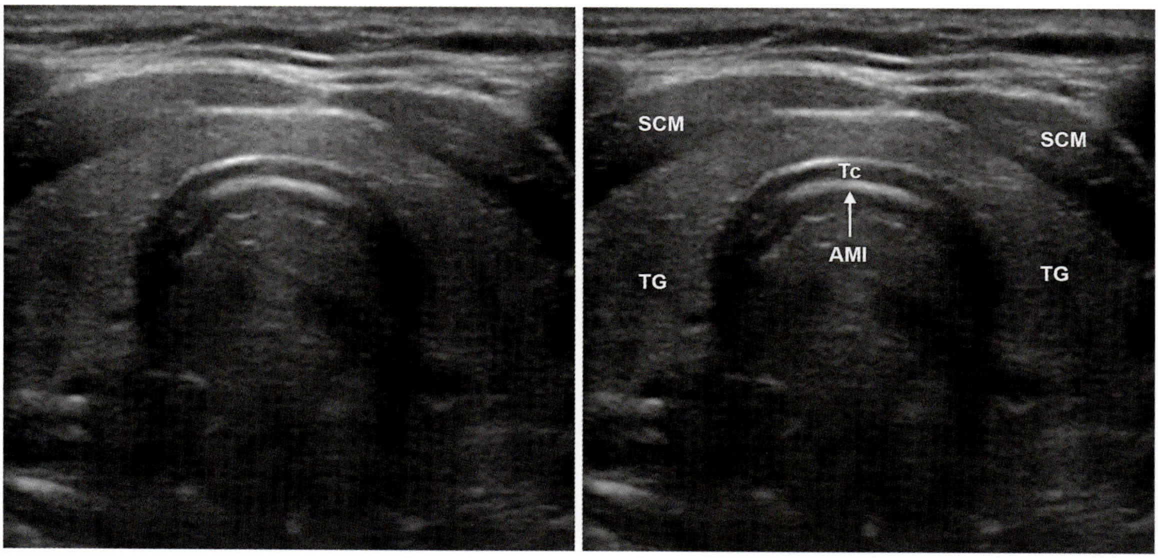

Fig. 11: Transverse view of trachea showing as "inverted U-shaped" structure. (AMI: air-mucosal interface; SCM: sternocleidomastoid muscle; Tc: tracheal cartilage; TG: thyroid gland)

location. This is called the "double bubble sign" **(Fig. 13)**. The absence of these signs indirectly confirms the correct placement of the endotracheal tube (ETT) inside the trachea. Esophageal placement of ETT can thus be recognized before the initiation of artificial ventilation. This is especially important in patients with full stomach such as in trauma settings.

- On the other hand, a direct sign of tracheal intubation is the "bullet sign", in which a single A-M interface with comet tail artifact

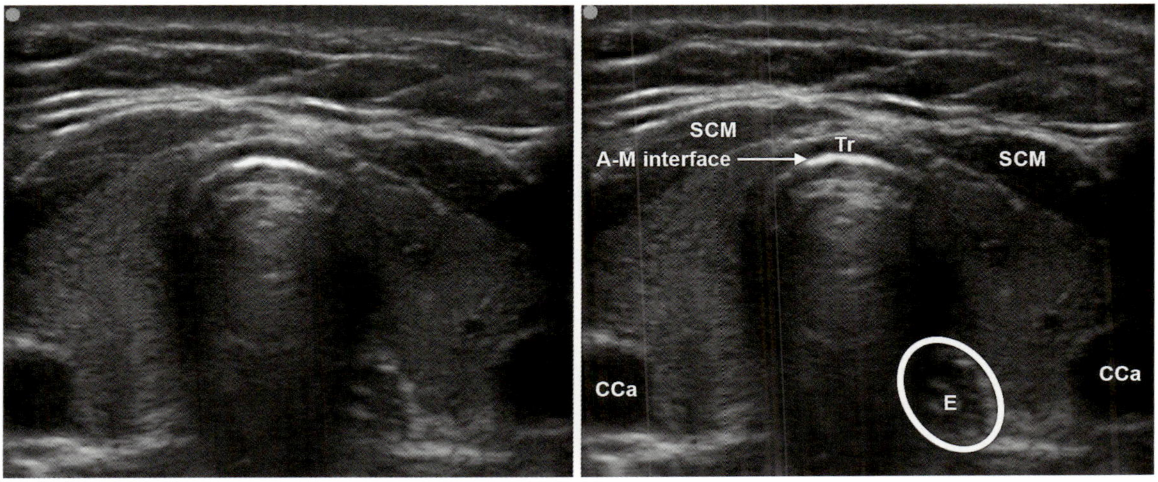

Fig. 12: Suprasternal transverse view showing esophagus in left posterior-lateral position. (CCa: common carotid artery; E: esophagus; SCM: sternocleidomastoid muscle; Tr: tracheal ring)

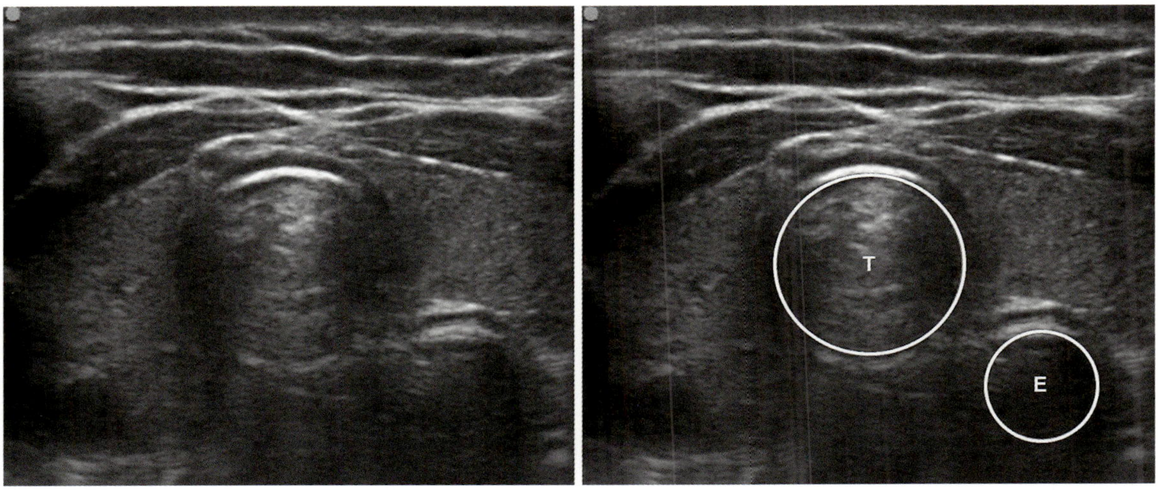

Fig. 13: Double bubble sign in suprasternal view depicting esophageal intubation. (E: esophageal lumen; T: tracheal lumen)

and posterior shadowing is observed. Movement can also be observed in the trachea as the ETT passes across the probe, called the "snowstorm sign". However, in 16% of the patients, the esophagus is located directly posterior to the trachea.[3]

- Adding lung ultrasound with positive lung-sliding sign to this method contributes to the diagnostic accuracy of endotracheal intubation and also helps to rule out endobronchial placement of ETT.

▪ *Identification of cricothyroid membrane:*
  - A cricothyroidotomy, although infrequent, is a lifesaving procedure that is used when other methods of accessing the airway fail, cannot intubate, cannot oxygenate

scenarios. It involves making an incision in the CTM and inserting a tube to establish an airway, i.e., surgical cricothyroidotomy or inserting a large bore cannula for emergent ventilation.

- Whether surgical or needle, cricothyroidotomy required identification of the CTM. The standard method of localizing CTM by palpating in the midline is not always successful, subsequently leading to the failure of cricothyroidotomy.It is especially challenging in obese patients or patients with abnormal neck anatomy.[4]
- Ultrasound facilitates prior identification and marking of the midpoint of the CTM in such situations.
- Kristensen et al. described two techniques to identify CTM. Commonly used, one is longitudinal or "string of pearl technique" and the other is transverse or "TACA (thyroid cartilage-airline-cricoid cartilage-airline) technique".[5]
- In the *longitudinal technique*, the transducer is placed in the sagittal plane above the suprasternal notch and slides to cephalad. CTM can be seen as a longitudinal hyperechoic line connecting thyroid and cricoid cartilages with an A-M interface posterior to it.
- In the *TACA technique*, the transducer is placed in the transverse plane on the anterior neck at the estimated level of the thyroid cartilage and moved to identify the thyroid cartilage (T) as an inverted V-shaped structure. Now, the transducer is moved caudal to get CTM as a hyperechoic transverse bright line due to the A-M interface (A). Further sliding caudally, horseshoe-shaped hypoechoic cricoid cartilage (C) is sighted. Then the transducer moved back cranially to get the A-M interface (A) again. Here, the midpoint of CTM is identified and marked.

- *Airway anesthesia for awake fiber-optic intubation:*
  - Airway blocks are an essential prerequisite for awake fiber-optic intubation. Topical local anesthetic (LA) application of airway by nebulization, spraying and gargling, is not adequate to anesthetize the whole path.
  - Ultrasound-guided airway blocks supplement the topicalization, hence assisting the preparation of the airway.
  - The superior surface of vocal cords, supraglottic laryngeal structures, and the laryngeal surface of the epiglottic are supplied by the internal branch of the superior laryngeal nerve. It enters the airway through the thyrohyoid membrane near the greater cornu of the hyoid bone. Here, it is blocked by infiltrating the LA in the thyrohyoid membrane in the targeted tissue plane with the help of ultrasound.
  - The subglottic structures and trachea get the supply via the recurrent laryngeal nerve, which are anesthetized by injecting LA with a 22-G IV cannula via CTM that can be identified by ultrasound as described above **(Table 2)**.
- *Percutaneous dilatational tracheostomy (PCT):*
  - Airway ultrasound is utilized for identification of tracheal rings for correct location and safe placement of percutaneous tracheostomy avoiding pretracheal blood vessels in both elective and emergency situations.
  - Accurate identification of anterior neck structures can eliminate potential complications such as hemorrhage, tracheal stenosis, erosion into high mediastinal vessels, and injury to the thyroid isthmus.
  - Preprocedural ultrasound can be utilized to examine the pretracheal area to look

for tracheal midline, approximate level of tracheal cartilages, anterior jugular veins, thyroid isthmus, and vulnerable thyroid vessels, and any other aberrant vessels in the area of interest.
- It also allows the selection of tracheostomy tube size by measuring the internal diameter of the trachea.
- Real-time PCT helps to avoid trauma to the posterior wall of the trachea. It is especially beneficial in patients with distorted anatomy.

- *Airway ultrasound—other applications:*
  - The application of ultrasound is not limited but extended to airway management.
  - It is useful for predicting difficult laryngoscopy and intubation by taking various measurements, especially in obese patients.
  - It also helps in the prediction of ETT size by assessing the narrowest diameter of the cricoid lumen.
  - Recently Difficult Airway Evaluation with Sonography (DARES) protocol has been described by Lin et al. (2023) to evaluate for difficult laryngoscopy.[4]
  - Identification of vocal cord palsy, epiglottitis, maxillary sinusitis, and laryngeal injury are also feasible.
  - Other applications include assessing laryngeal edema, predicting post-extubation stridor, and detecting the correct position of the laryngeal mask airway.

CONCLUSION

- Despite the remarkable utility of ultrasound in elective and emergency airway management, airway ultrasound is not without limitations.
- Ultrasound waves cannot pass through the air, so deeper structures are not visualized.
- In some conditions, such as subcutaneous emphysema, posterior laryngeal injury, and age-related calcification of cartilages, artifacts may interfere with imaging.
- Image acquisition and interpretation are operator-dependent but have a steep learning curve.

REFERENCES

1. Kolli S, Singh M. POCUS spotlight: airway. ASRA News. 2021;46(3).
2. Chowdhury AR, Punj J, Pandey R, Darlong V, Sinha R, Bhoi D. Ultrasound is a reliable and faster tool for confirmation of endotracheal intubation compared to chest auscultation and capnography when performed by novice anaesthesia residents - A prospective controlled clinical trial. Saudi J Anaesth. 2020;14(1):15-21.
3. Tsung JW, Fenster D, Kessler DO, Novik J. Dynamic anatomic relationship of the esophagus and trachea on sonography: implications for endotracheal tube confirmation in children. J Ultrasound Med. 2012;31(9):1365-70.
4. Lin J, Bellinger R, Shedd A, Wolfshohl J, Walker J, Healy J, et al. Point-of-Care Ultrasound in Airway Evaluation and Management: A Comprehensive Review. Diagnostics (Basel). 2023;13(9):1541.
5. Kristensen MS, Teoh WH, Rudolph SS. Ultrasonographic identification of the cricothyroid membrane: Best evidence, techniques, and clinical impact. Br J Anaesth. 2016;117 Suppl 1:i39–i48.

CHAPTER 4

Lung Ultrasound

Alka Verma, Divya Srivastava, Pallav Singh

WHAT YOU WILL LEARN IN THIS CHAPTER?

A. Application of lung ultrasound (LUS) in emergency department (ED) and intensive care units (ICUs)

B. Differentiating normal and abnormal images

C. Recognition of common lung pathologies on ultrasound (USG)

INTRODUCTION

The ultrasound (USG) has gradually emerged as an important bedside tool in diagnosing pulmonary ailments, monitoring the effects of treatment given and guiding therapeutic interventions. Until 1989, USG was considered a useless modality as far as lung scans were concerned, as the air-filled organ did not allow passage of ultrasonic waves. A healthy lung is not visible in USG scanning. Indeed, the lung USG is primarily based on the interpretation of artifacts produced by the reflection of sound waves from healthy as well as unhealthy tissue. Pleural line, pleural effusions, and consolidated lung, however, are visible and easily recognized.

Since even the semiquantitative assessment of B-lines is subjected to operator, hardware, and image settings variability, the final interpretation must be an amalgam of the patient's clinical situation and other imaging done.

WHY DO ULTRASONIC SCANNING OF LUNGS?

Lung ultrasound (LUS) has crept into multiple settings as an important everyday tool and is rightly labeled as the "stethoscopes" of modern physicians. It can be performed at the bedside of the patients, and is reliable, repeatable, and provides immediate information on the condition of the organ scanned. **Table 1** deals with the uses of LUS in hospital settings.

PREPARATIONS FOR SCAN

Machine preparation: Irrespective of the make of the USG machine, the scan setting is kept at "lung scan". If the "lung scan" option is not available, care must be taken to deactivate the artifact-erasing software for proper interpretation of the scan.

No specific probe is recommended, but most used probes are phased array (2–8 MHz) or microconvex (3.5–8 MHz) as it enables scanning to greater depths and prevents repeated changing of probes. For assessing superficial aspects of the lungs, such as pleural movements and pneumothorax, the linear probe is used. It is particularly helpful in diagnosing pneumothorax. Both 2D and M-mode are used to scan each area.

Patient preparation: The machine and the clinician stand on the right side of the patient by convention. It is important to explain the procedure to all conscious patients before baring their chests for the scan. The patients must also be warned of the cold feel of USG jelly. The patient is made to lie with hands outstretched to enable scanning of the anterior zone **(Fig. 1)**. To enhance the scan of lateral and posterior zones,

TABLE 1: Uses of lung ultrasound.

Hospital settings	*Utility*	
Emergency department	• Aid in diagnosis	• As part of quick scan for patients presenting with dyspnea and acute respiratory failure
	• Monitoring	• Effect of immediate management done
Trauma	• Diagnosis	• Bedside quick diagnosis of pneumothorax, hemothorax, rib fractures, pulmonary contusions, and chest wall hematomas
	• Aid in intervention	• Ultrasound (USG)-guided chest drain insertion
Intensive care unit (ICU)	• Aid in monitoring	• Day-to-day examination of lung conditions, much like auscultation
	• Patients on mechanical ventilation	• *Monitoring effect of treatment and guide the management:* Development of any iatrogenic pathology due to mechanical ventilation
	• Aid in diagnosing	
	• Aid in intervention	• US-guided drain of loculated pleural collections

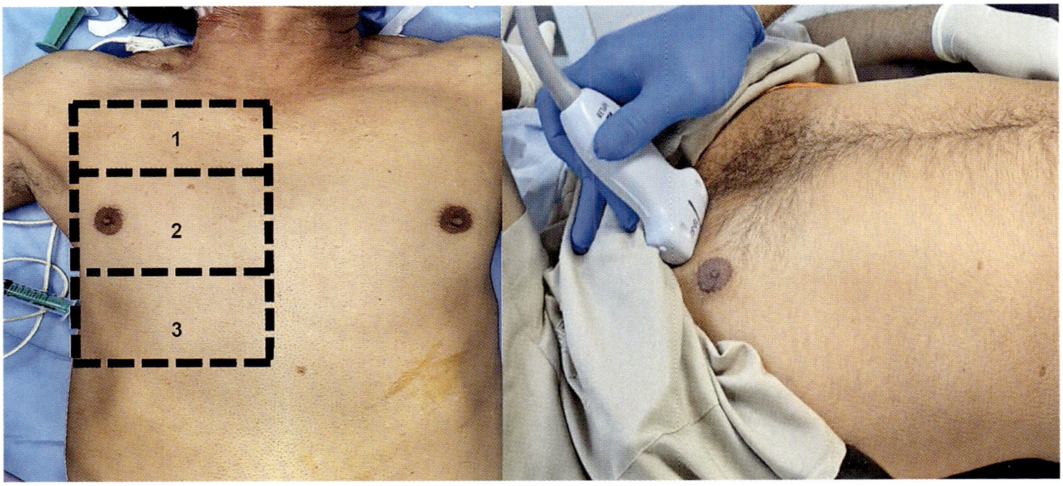

Fig. 1: Anterior zones of lung scan, 18 scan zone.

the patient is tilted laterally with the help of an assistant **(Fig. 2)**. The marker of the probe is placed cranially.

PROBE POSITIONING AND SURFACE ANATOMY

Images are obtained in six lung zones: Anterior, lateral, and posterior zones on either side to cover the entire lungs **(Fig. 3)**.

- *Anterior zone:* It covers the anterior aspect of upper, middle, and lower lung lobes on right side and anterior aspect of upper lobe on left side.
- *Lateral zone:* It scans the lateral part of upper lobes, parts of lower and middle lobe on right side, and lateral part of lower lobe on left side.
- *Posterior zone:* It covers the posterior aspect of both upper and lower lobes on either sides.

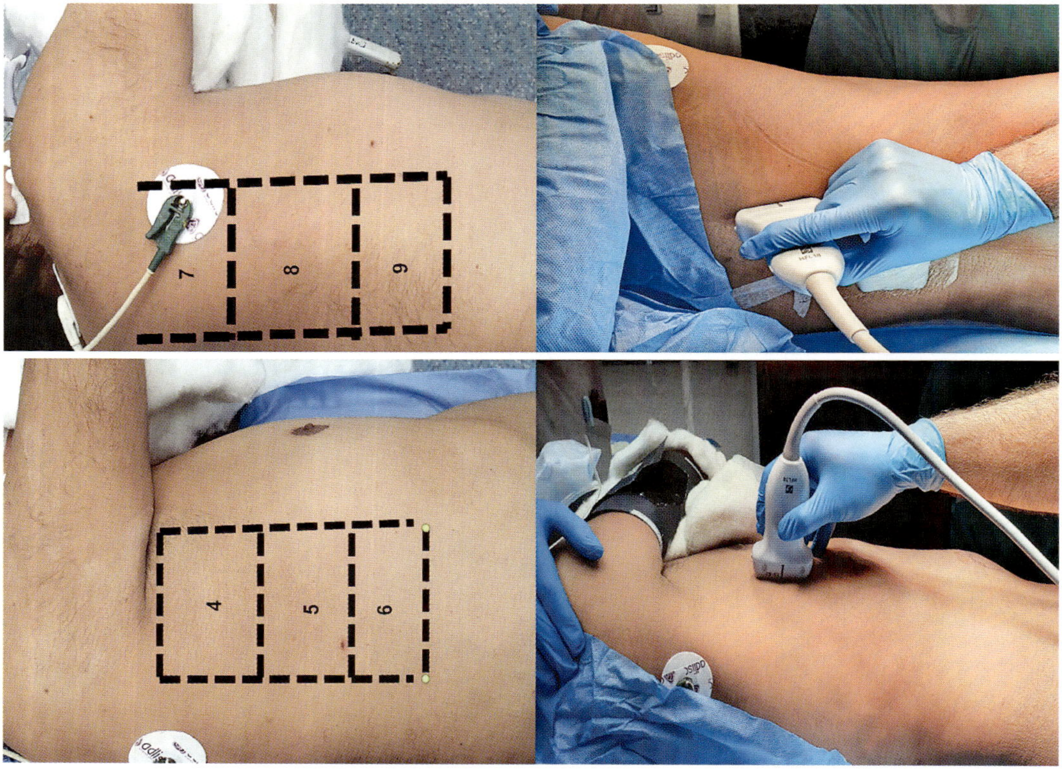

Fig. 2: Lateral and posterior zone scans require tilting of the patient, 18 scan zones.

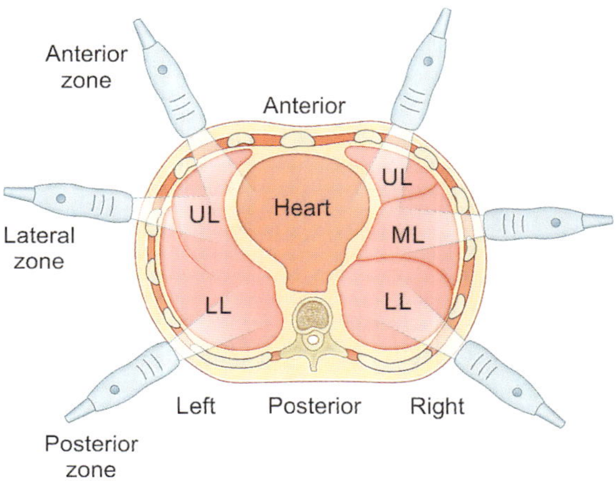

Fig. 3: Surface anatomy and lung lobes.

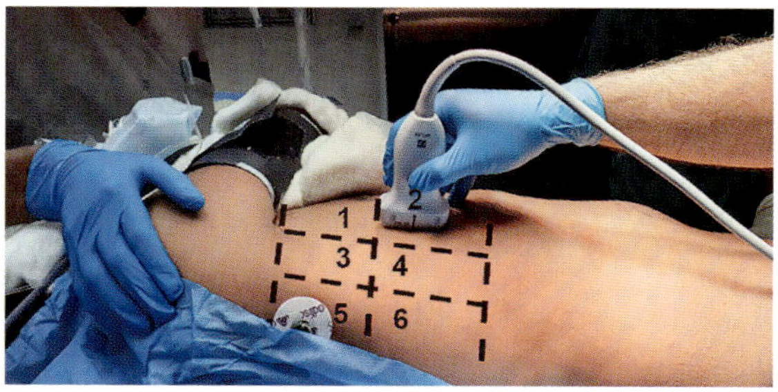

Fig. 4: 12 scan zones.

Some practitioners scan two sections: (1) Upper and (2) lower in each zone, creating a total of 12 scan areas **(Fig. 4)**, while few others prefer scanning three interspaces in each zone creating 18 scan areas **(Figs. 1 and 2)**.[1] The literature is crammed with protocols for LUS; BLUE, RADIUS, FALLS, FLUID, and ETUDES. No matter what protocol is followed, it is important to scan the entire chest thoroughly before concluding on the findings.

NORMAL LUNG INTERPRETATION

Lung ultrasound images are basically artifacts created by the movement of sound waves through acoustically different subcutaneous tissue and air-filled lungs. Each area of the lung is scanned to confirm the presence or absence of these artifacts; lung sliding sign, A- and B-lines, and air bronchograms.

Bat wing sign: The first placement of the probe is longitudinal between the two ribs. The probe is then tilted on either side to obtain an image of dark rib shadows of upper and lower ribs with a shinning hyperechoic pleural line in-between. This happens when the probe is perfectly perpendicular to the pleura. **Figure 5** shows what is classically known as "bat wing sign", determining the proper placement of the USG probe.

Once an area is localized in a longitudinal scan the probe is rotated transversely to get a better view of the pleura and its related artifacts without hindrance from rib shadows.

A-lines: Air-filled alveoli in the lungs scatter most of the sound waves. The parietal pleura, however, is visualized as a shiny white line called the pleural line. Healthy alveolar tissue beyond this is not seen. Instead, parallel horizontal hyperechoic lines that are reverberations of the pleural line are visualized. The distance between two A-lines is the same as the distance between the pleura and the USG probe. These lines are called A-lines **(Fig. 6)**.

Lung sliding sign: As the lungs expand and contract with each breath the parietal and visceral pleura slide on each other. The impression given by movement of visceral pleura over parietal pleura on USG imaging is like waves produced in a

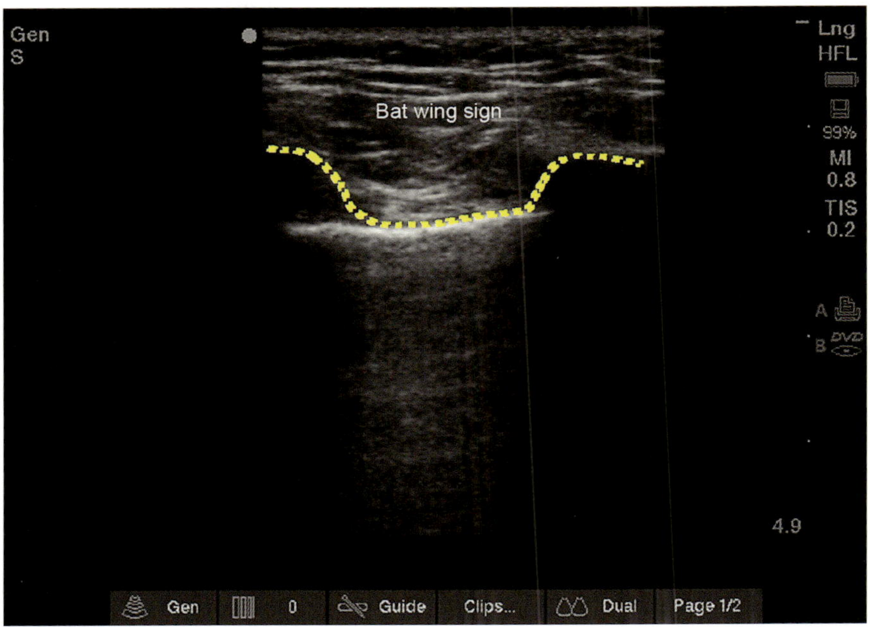

Fig. 5: Bat wing sign.

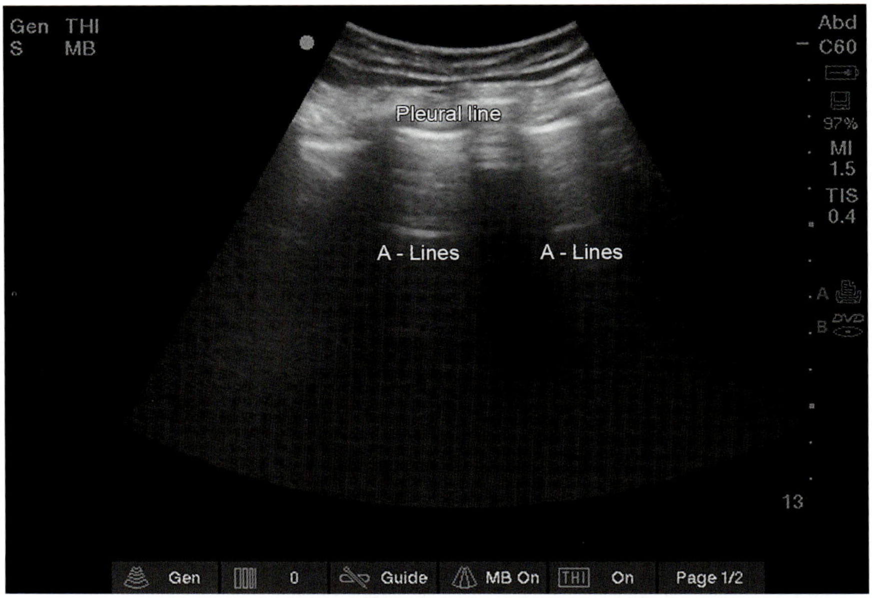

Fig. 6: A-lines.

curtain. This is called "lung sliding sign". Presence of this sign ensures presence of ventilation in the scanned zone. Absence of lung sliding points toward a diagnosis of pneumothorax or hyperinflated lungs.

Seashore sign: When M-mode is placed in the center of the pleural line, a "seashore sign" appears on the screen. The tissue above the pleural line is seen as static, linear lines while due to the scattering of sound waves by lung tissue below the pleura, sand-like granules are seen below the pleural line. The image resembles that of a sandy shore and sea junction, hence the name. Its presence again is interpreted as a normally ventilated lung zone **(Fig. 7)**.

Lung pulse: Pulses generated by the beating heart are normally transmitted to pleura. In the absence of lung sliding, movement of the pleural line may still be visible synchronous to the heartbeat. Though similar to the lung sliding sign prima facie, its coinciding with heartbeats helps in differentiation. This indicates that the lung zone is not being ventilated; bronchial intubation, lung contusion, hyperinflation of lung zone, or early atelectasis.

B-lines: The first International Consensus Conference on LUS defined B-lines as "discrete laser-like vertical hyperechoic reverberation artifacts that arise from the pleural line and extend to the bottom of the screen without fading".[2] These lines move synchronously to the pleural lines. Increased density in interstitial spaces generates these lines. The presence of up to three discrete lines in each zone is considered normal. An increase in their number or coalescence of B-lines is an indication of deteriorating lung aeration and presence of an underlying pathology.

LUNG SCORING FOR SEMIQUANTITATIVE ASSESSMENT

Several LUS scoring systems are available. BLUE protocol or a twelve-zone examination is most

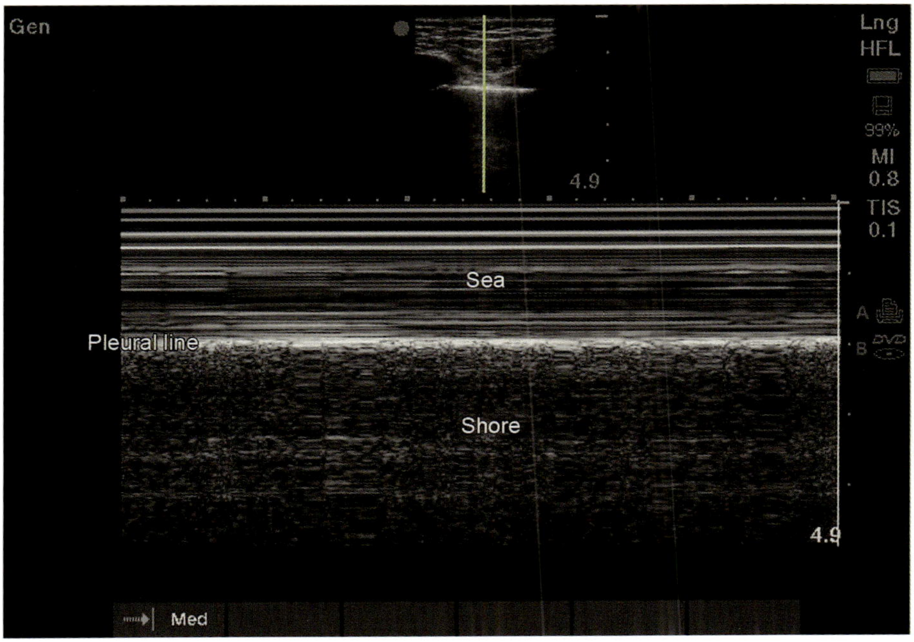

Fig. 7: Seashore sign.

TABLE 2: Semiquantitative assessment of lung zones.

Score	*Image*	*Interpretation*
0	A-lines with lung sliding or 1–3 B-lines visible	Normal aeration
1	Greater than 3 B-lines either spaced or coalescent. Subpleural consolidation <50% scan area	Moderate loss of aeration
2	Coalescent B lines, subpleural consolidation >50% of scan area	Severe loss of aeration
3	Tissue-like pattern/ visualization of consolidated lung/hepatization of lung	Complete absence of aeration

used by critical care experts.[3] Each zone is scored from 0 to 3 depending on images obtained in the region **(Table 2 and Figs. 8A to D)**. Total LUS ranges from 0 to 36 and helps in monitoring and guiding the treatment of the patients.

LUNG PATHOLOGIES ON ULTRASOUND

- *Pneumothorax:*
  - Pneumothorax occurs when air accumulates within pleural space due to disruption of the visceral and parietal pleura.
  - *Ultrasound findings in pneumothorax:*
    - *Absence of lung sliding*: The shimmering effect of the pleural line, due to gliding of pleural layers, is absent due to air in the space.
    - *Absent B-lines:* B-lines are vertical lines that arise from the pleura and move with respiration, usually seen in normal lungs. In pneumothorax, these lines are absent.
    - *Presence of the "barcode" or "stratosphere" sign on M-mode:* When M-mode is used on the pleural line, a normal lung will show a "seashore" pattern due to

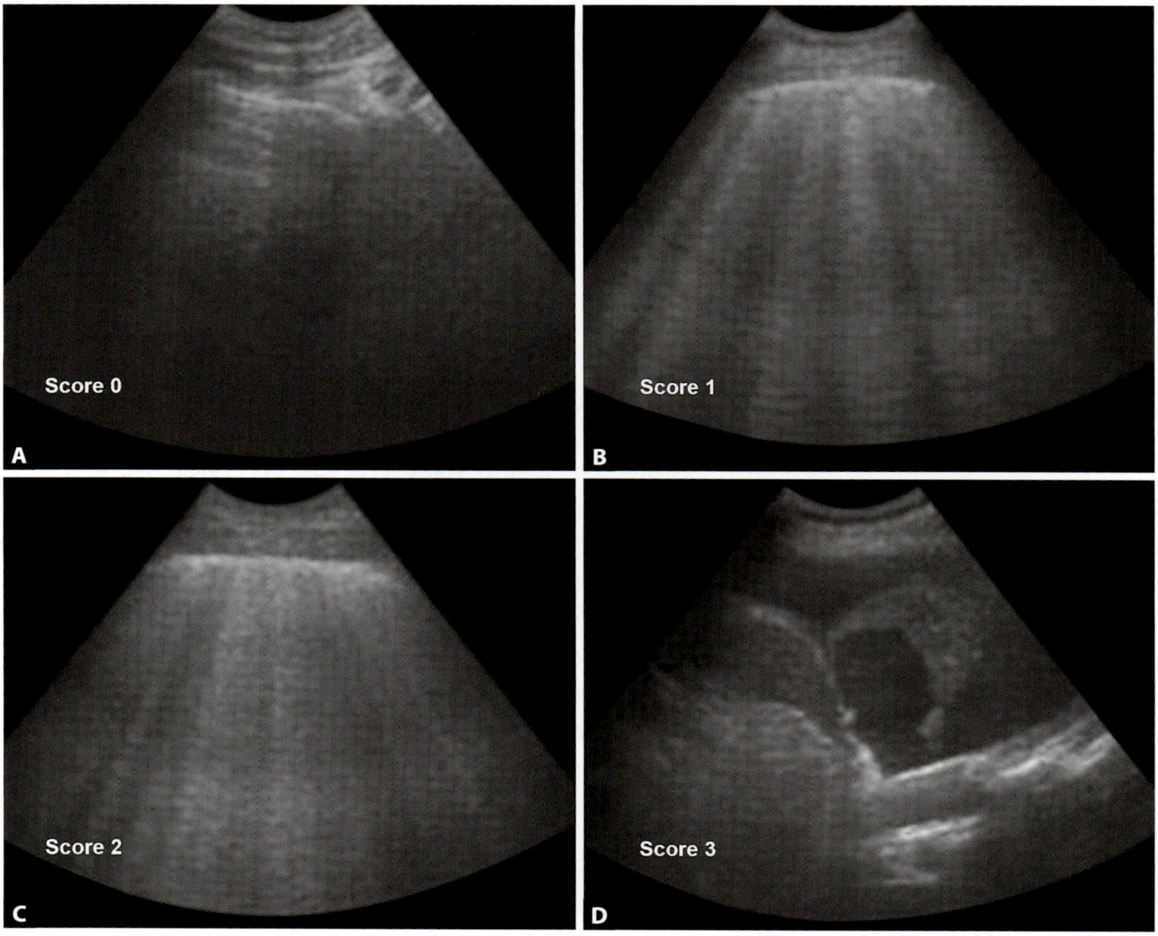

Figs. 8A to D: (A) Presence of lung sliding with A-lines or fewer than two isolated B-lines; (B) Well-defined B-lines; (C) Multiple coalescent B-lines; (D) Lung consolidation.

movement, while a pneumothorax will display a "barcode" or "stratosphere" pattern, indicating no lung movement **(Fig. 9)**.

- *Lung point sign:* The lung point is the area where the pneumothorax starts and the lung adheres to the pleura again. This is a highly specific sign for pneumothorax. The presence of a lung point is 100% specific for confirming a diagnosis of pneumothorax.
- *Pleural line shift:* In some cases, the pleural line may appear shifted or discontinuous due to air in the pleural space.

- *Pleural effusion:*
  - In various conditions, such as heart failure, infection, malignancy, or inflammation, abnormal accumulation of fluid occurs in the pleural space, known as pleural effusion, which can impair lung expansion.

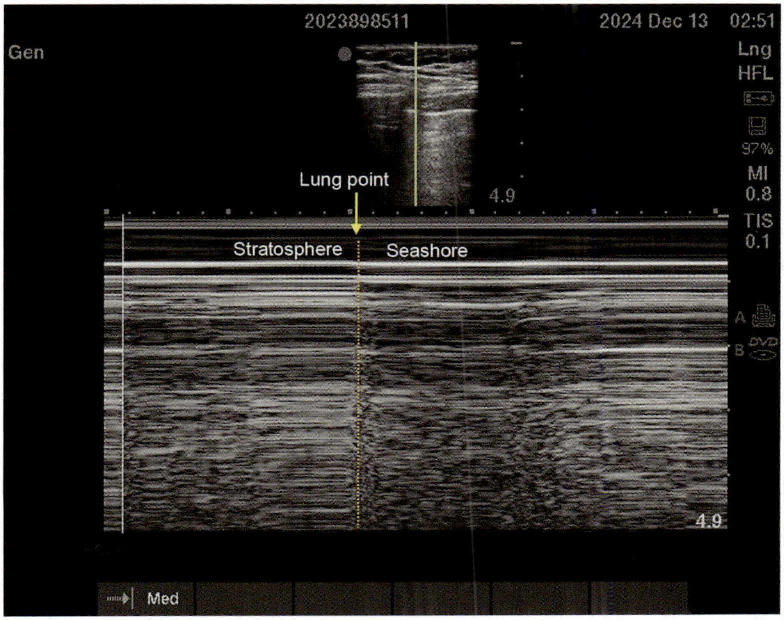

Fig. 9: Lung point (pneumothorax).

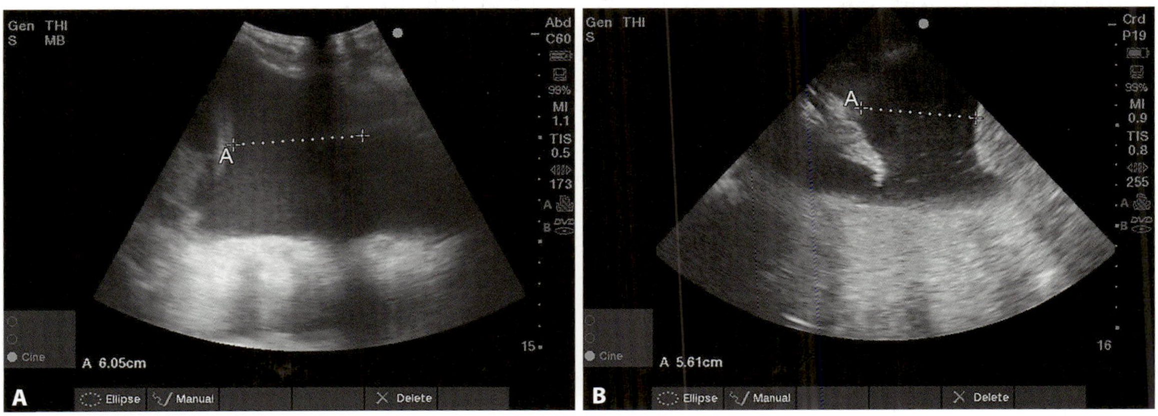

Figs. 10A and B: Fluid appears as a dark (anechoic) or less echogenic (hypoechoic) area in the pleural space.

- *Ultrasound findings in pleural effusion* ***(Figs. 10 to 14)****:*
  - *Anechoic or hypoechoic area:* Fluid appears as a dark (anechoic) or less echogenic (hypoechoic) area in the pleural space **(Figs. 10A and B)**.
  - *Floating lung or lung flapping or jellyfish sign:* The lung may appear to "float" or move within the fluid, resembling the movement of a jellyfish with respiration **(Figs. 11A and B)**.
  - *Spine sign:* The thoracic spine becomes visible above the diaphragm due to the presence of fluid, which acts as an acoustic window **(Figs. 12A and B)**.

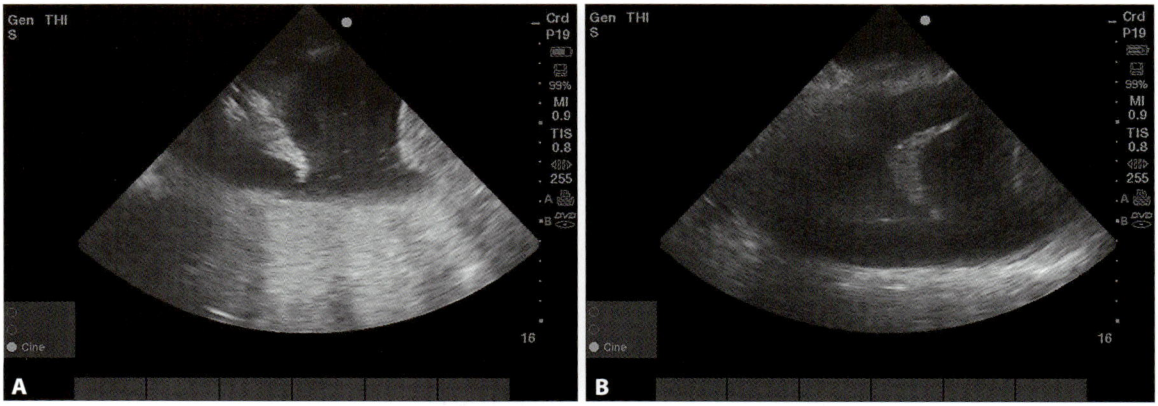

Figs. 11A and B: Jelly fish sign.

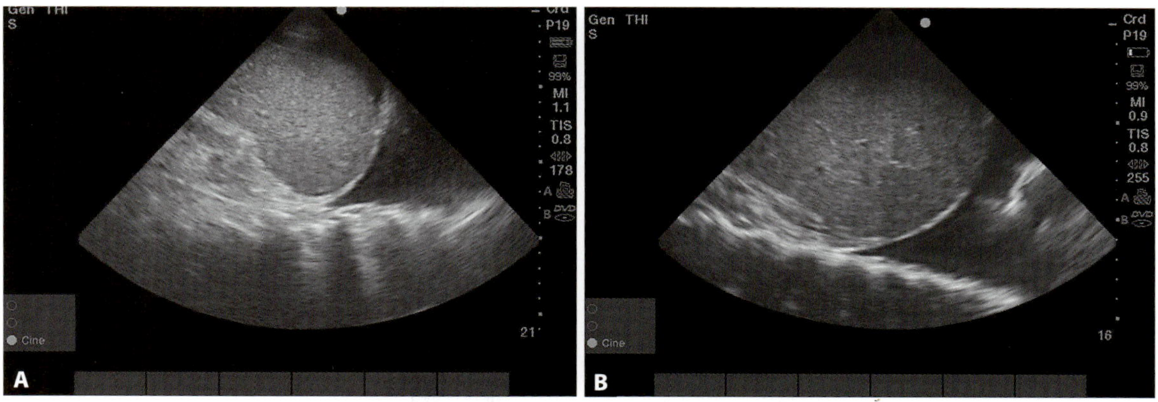

Figs. 12A and B: Pleural effusion spine sign.

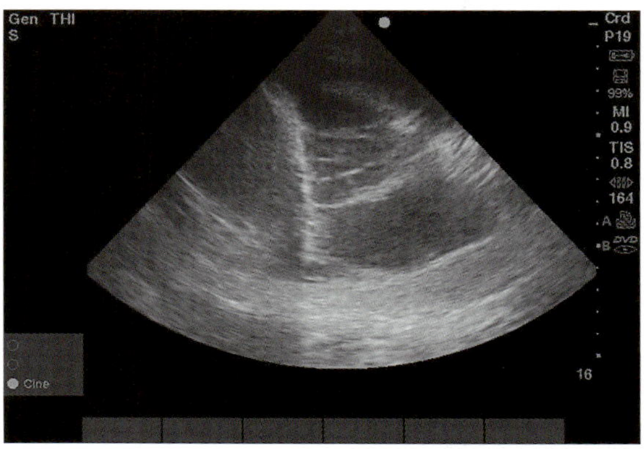

Fig. 13: Septated pleural effusion.

- *Sinusoid sign:* On M-mode, the pleural fluid between the parietal and visceral pleura shows a sinusoidal pattern, confirming the presence of free fluid.
- *Mirror image artifact:* This occurs when the liver or spleen appears to extend above the diaphragm, a sign of fluid in the pleural space reflecting sound waves.
- *Diaphragm flattening or inversion:* The diaphragm may appear flattened or inverted due to pressure from a large effusion.

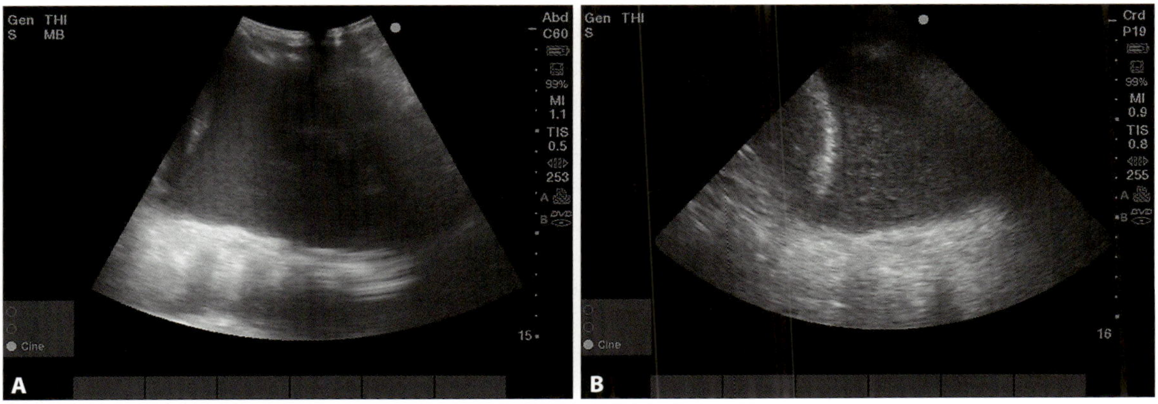

Figs. 14A and B: *Hematocrit sign:* Exudative pleural effusion: spontaneous ECHO contrast (SEC).

- *Atelectatic lung:* Echogenic lung tissue may be visualized as compressed or consolidated within the effusion, indicating atelectasis.
- *Pleural thickening and septated pleural effusion:* In some cases, thickening of the pleura and septated pleural effusion are observed, which may suggest an exudative effusion or underlying pleural pathology **(Fig. 13)**.
- *Hematocrit sign:* Separation of fluid and cellular contents of effusion is seen in hemothorax or exudative pleural effusion. An anechoic shadow of fluid and heterogeneously hypoechoic shadow of the cellular component is visible on LUS (**Figs. 14A and B**).

- *Pneumonia:*
  - Pneumonia is defined as an infection within the lung parenchyma that leads to consolidation, visible as a hypoechoic or echogenic area within the lung tissue.
  - Pneumonia disrupts normal aeration, resulting in a "hepatization" appearance, where the affected lung area resembles the echotexture of the liver.
  - *Ultrasound findings in pneumonia:*
    - *Dynamic air bronchograms:* Moving, bright spots within the consolidated area, representing air within bronchi.
    - *Pleural line abnormalities:* The pleural line overlying the consolidated area may be thickened or irregular.
    - *B-lines:* Vertical, hyperechoic lines that radiate from the pleural line and extend deep into the lung, often seen surrounding the consolidation.
    - *Shred sign:* The irregular or shredded border of the consolidated lung, indicating alveolar involvement **(Fig. 15)**.
    - *Lung consolidation:* The infected lung tissue appears as a solid area, often with hyperechoic punctate areas that represent trapped air **(Fig. 16)**.
- *Cardiogenic pulmonary edema:*
  - In cardiogenic pulmonary edema, fluid accumulates in the lungs due to increased pressure in the pulmonary capillaries, typically resulting from left-sided heart failure.
  - When the heart's left ventricle cannot effectively pump blood forward, pressure builds up backward in the left atrium and

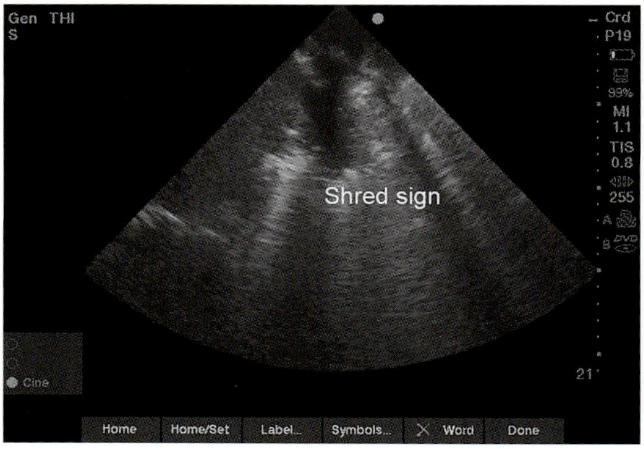

Fig. 15: Shred sign.

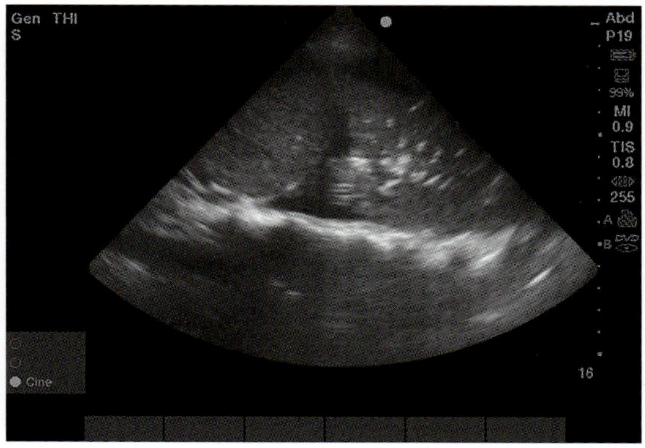

Fig. 16: Consolidation.

pulmonary veins, forcing fluid out of the capillaries and into the alveolar spaces and lung interstitium.

- *Ultrasound findings in cardiogenic pulmonary edema include:*
  - *Multiple B-lines:* Vertical, hyperechoic lines arising from the pleural line and extending deep into the lung field, resembling "comet tails." In cardiogenic pulmonary edema, multiple B-lines appear diffusely across lung fields, indicating interstitial fluid.
  - *Thickened pleural line:* The pleural line may appear thickened due to fluid accumulation in the interstitial spaces.
  - *Subpleural consolidations:* Small and patchy hypoechoic areas near the pleural surface, representing areas of lung tissue collapse or micro-consolidations due to fluid overload.
  - *Pleural effusion:* Often present as a secondary finding, typically in the dependent areas of the lung, and appears as an anechoic or hypoechoic area between the lung and chest wall.
  - *"White lung" appearance:* When B-lines are numerous and close together, they can create a near-continuous bright or "white" appearance on USG, indicating significant interstitial edema.
  - *Absence of lung sliding:* In severe cases, reduced or absent lung sliding may be seen due to the stiffness of fluid-filled lungs.

- *Acute respiratory distress syndrome (ARDS):*
  - ARDS is a severe, inflammatory lung condition characterized by acute onset of widespread alveolar damage and respiratory failure.
  - ARDS shows specific signs due to the severe, diffuse alveolar, and interstitial damage it causes. These USG findings help to differentiate ARDS from other causes of respiratory distress, such as cardiogenic pulmonary edema.
  - *Ultrasound findings in ARDS include:*
    - *Multiple B-lines (comet tails) in patchy distribution:* Unlike cardiogenic pulmonary edema, B-lines in ARDS are often unevenly distributed, with both spared and affected areas. This pattern reflects the heterogeneous involvement of the lung.
    - *Thickened and irregular pleural line:* The pleural line in ARDS often appears thickened and irregular, indicating damage to the alveolar-capillary barrier.

- *Subpleural consolidations:* Small, hypoechoic areas beneath the pleura, reflecting areas of alveolar collapse or consolidation.
- *Lung sliding:* Lung sliding may be diminished in areas of severe consolidation or atelectasis but is generally preserved in other regions.
- *"Spared areas":* Unlike cardiogenic edema, ARDS often has areas of normal lung interspersed with diseased lung, creating a patchy pattern on USG.
- *Larger consolidations and air bronchograms:* More extensive consolidations with air bronchograms (air-filled bronchi within consolidated areas) may be visible, especially in the dependent regions of the lung.
- *Pleural effusion:* Less common in ARDS than in cardiogenic edema, but small effusions may be present, particularly if associated with fluid overload from treatment.

- *Chronic obstructive pulmonary disease (COPD):*
  - COPD primarily reflects hyperinflation and air trapping rather than specific structural changes, given that COPD affects the lung's ability to expand and contract normally.
  - *Ultrasound findings in COPD include:*
    - *Prominent A-lines:* Horizontal, repetitive lines below the pleural line, representing normal air artifacts due to hyperinflation and trapped air. A-lines are the dominant artifact in COPD and indicate a lack of significant lung interstitial involvement.
    - *Reduced or absent B-lines:* B-lines (vertical artifacts) are generally absent in stable COPD, as they suggest interstitial fluid, which is not a feature of COPD unless there is coexisting heart failure or infection.
    - *Thickened and irregular pleural line:* Chronic inflammation and structural remodeling in COPD can cause pleural irregularities, seen as a thickened and sometimes interrupted pleural line on USG.
    - *Decreased lung sliding:* Lung sliding, a shimmer-like movement of the pleura during respiration, may be reduced or subtle in severe COPD due to air trapping, which restricts lung movement against the chest wall.
    - *Diaphragmatic flattening and limited motion:* COPD often leads to diaphragmatic flattening and reduced diaphragmatic excursion, which can be visualized on USG. Limited diaphragm movement is associated with hyperinflation and air trapping, particularly in severe cases.
    - *Bullae or large air spaces:* In advanced COPD, large air-filled spaces (bullae) may be present, which can appear as areas without normal lung sliding and without artifacts (anechoic regions).
- *Pulmonary embolism (PE):*
  - PE refers to the obstruction of pulmonary arteries by a blood clot, which can lead to signs of lung infarction or associated complications rather than direct visualization of the embolism itself, as USG cannot directly visualize clots in the pulmonary arteries.
  - However, certain indirect USG findings may suggest PE, especially when combined with clinical suspicion and other imaging modalities, such as echocardiography and Doppler USG for deep vein thrombosis (DVT).
  - *Ultrasound findings in PE include:*
    - *Wedge-shaped and pleural-based consolidations:* Hypoechoic, triangular

areas adjacent to the pleura, often in the lung periphery. These may represent pulmonary infarcts caused by emboli obstructing blood flow.

- *Absence of B-lines:* In affected areas, there is often a lack of B-lines (which indicate interstitial fluid), as PE typically leads to infarction rather than interstitial fluid accumulation.
- *Peripheral hypoechoic lesions:* Small, round, or wedge-shaped hypoechoic lesions with or without air bronchograms may be seen in the lung periphery, indicating infarction.
- *Pleural effusion:* A small, unilateral pleural effusion may be present, often on the side of the embolism, due to local inflammation or infarction.
- *Right ventricular dysfunction on cardiac USG:* A common finding associated with PE, visible on echocardiography, includes right ventricular dilation and dysfunction, indicating increased pulmonary pressure and strain due to embolic obstruction.

LIMITATIONS

Lung ultrasound is a highly operator-dependent technique. Since LUS is mainly interpretation of artifacts, the images obtained are influenced by the selection of probe, depth, and gain settings. Careful interpretation of scans is thus required to prevent false negatives and false positives in the diagnosis and monitoring of patients. There are certain conditions when LUS fails to be of help **(Table 3)**.

TABLE 3: Limitations of LUS.

Condition	*Reason*
Subcutaneous emphysema	Ultrasound waves are unable to pass through air interfaces, LUS fails to come to aid in patients with subcutaneous emphysema
Heavy body habitus	Obese and heavily built patients may have obscured lung window due to increased depth of viscera
Asthma/COPD/ pulmonary embolism	Imaging same as in normal lung. Diagnosis is not possible by LUS alone

(COPD: chronic obstructive pulmonary disease; LUS: lung ultrasound)

CONCERNS

For practical purposes, routine and frequent use of USG for monitoring and guiding the management is considered safe for the patients. Animal models have shown incidences of pulmonary capillary hemorrhage, raising concerns of safety of its use in monitoring the progress of diseases. Such incidences, however, have not been replicated in human subjects.

CONCLUSION

Lung ultrasound has rapidly gained acceptance in emergency departments, semi-ICUs, ICUs, and even wards for bedside assessment of patients. It can aid in diagnosing etiology behind hypoxemia in up to 90% cases.[4]

A thorough training though is essential before one starts using USG machine for routine lung scans in their settings. Rocca et al.[5], have rightly pointed out that beginners in LUS are able to identify A-lines, B-lines, consolidation, and pleural effusion, a further experience enables one to recognize sliding signs, lung pulse, lung point, interpretation of air bronchograms, and quantification of pleural effusions. Advanced and expert LUS users are able to compute LUS scores and use them to guide management and ventilation strategies. The number of scans needed or the duration of experience required to reach to that level has not yet been defined. Nevertheless, LUS continues to be an important tool in our everyday practice.

REFERENCES

1. Manson WC, Hogg RM. (2022). POCUS Spotlight: Lung Ultrasound. [online] Available from https://www.asra.com/news-publications/asra-newsletter/newsletter-item/asra-news/2022/02/07/point-of-care-ultrasound-spotlight-lung-ultrasound [Last accessed August, 2025].
2. Volpicelli G, Elbarbary M, Blaivas M, Lichtenstein DA, Mathis G, Kirkpatrick AW, et al. International Liaison Committee on Lung Ultrasound (ILC-LUS) for International Consensus Conference on Lung Ultrasound (ICC-LUS). International evidence-based recommendations for point-of-care lung ultrasound. Intensive Care Med. 2012;38(4):577-91.
3. Chiumello D, Mongodi S, Algieri I, Vergani GL, Orlando A, Via G, et al. Assessment of lung aeration and recruitment by ct scan and ultrasound in acute respiratory distress syndrome patients. Crit Care Med. 2018;46(11):1761-8.
4. Lichtenstein DA, Mezière GA. Relevance of lung ultrasound in the diagnosis of acute respiratory failure: the BLUE protocol. Chest. 2008;134(1):117-25. Erratum in: Chest. 2013;144(2):721.
5. Rocca E, Zanza C, Longhitano Y, Piccolella F, Romenskaya T, Racca F, et al. Lung ultrasound in critical care and emergency medicine: Clinical Review. Adv Respir Med. 2023;91(3):203-23.

CHAPTER 5

Transthoracic Echocardiography

Amit Anand, Subhankar Paul

WHAT YOU WILL LEARN IN THIS CHAPTER?

A. Different echocardiographic windows:
  - ♦ Left parasternal window (PLAX, PSAX)
  - ♦ Apical four chamber including two-, three-, and five-chamber view
  - ♦ Subcostal view
  - ♦ Suprasternal window

B. Assessment of left ventricular (LV) anatomy and function

C. Assessment of right ventricular (RV) anatomy and function

D. Pulmonary artery (PA) pressure assessment

E. Screening for aortic dissection

F. Inferior vena cava (IVC) measurement

G. Pericardial effusion and measurement with tamponade feature

INTRODUCTION

Transthoracic echocardiography (TTE) is a quick noninvasive cardiac imaging modality which uses ultrasound waves to evaluate heart and great vessels. First report of use of ultrasound for cardiovascular diagnosis was by Edler and Hertz in 1954.

WHY DO ECHOCARDIOGRAPHY IN EMERGENCY?

Common clinical situations where TTE can play a useful role in diagnosis and management of patients in emergency department.

- Chest pain
- Unexplained breathlessness
- Palpitation
- Undifferentiated shock
- Clinically heard murmurs
- Fluid status monitoring
- Postcardiac arrest
- Cyanotic patients
- Suspected infective endocarditis
- Prosthetic valve evaluation

MODALITIES OF ECHOCARDIOGRAPHY

We use multiple echocardiographic modalities to evaluate various aspects of cardiac function:

- Two-dimensional (2D) echocardiography
- M-mode (motion mode)
- *Doppler echocardiography:*
  - Color flow mapping (CFM)
  - Continuous wave (CW) Doppler
  - Pulsed wave (PW) Doppler
  - Tissue Doppler imaging (TDI)

PREPARATION FOR TRANSTHORACIC ECHOCARDIOGRAPHY

- *Patient position:* Semirecumbent position
- *Lie:* Patient lying on left side, head of patient slightly elevated

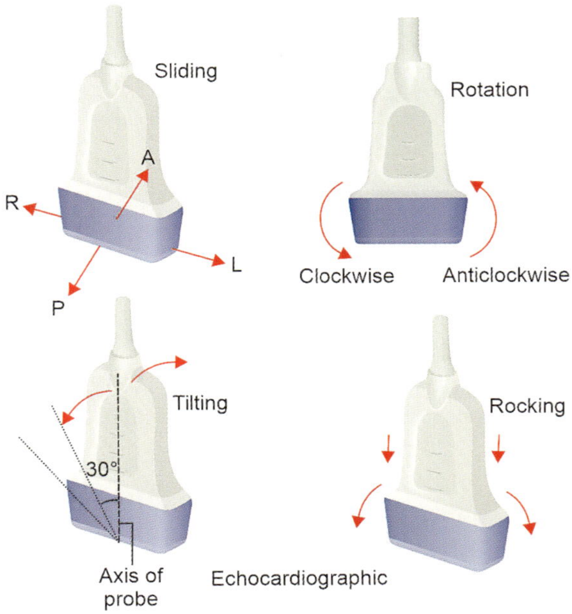

Fig. 1: Different probe maneuvers to obtain the best view. (A: anterior; P: posterior)

- *Left arm:* Under the head
- *Right arm:* Alongside the body [opens intercostal space (ICS)]
- Ideal examination is in expiration.
- *Probe:* 3–5 MHz probe
- *Medium:* Ultrasound jelly to be applied.
- *Echo machine placement:* Preferably on the right side of the patient, hold the probe with right hand and use left hand for machine keypad handling
- *Manipulations to obtain a good echocardiography window* ***(Fig. 1 and Table 1)***
  - Sliding
  - Tilting
  - Rotation
  - Rocking

OBTAINING THE ECHOCARDIOGRAPHIC VIEWS

Figures 2 and 3 summarize the different probe position with marker orientation to obtain different echocardiographic views. We would now summarize the different views and information we can receive from them in emergency echocardiography.

TABLE 1: Definition of various manipulations for best echocardiographic views.

Manipulation	*Definition*
Tilt	The transducer maintains same axis orientation to the heart but moves to a different imaging plane
Rotate	The transducer maintains a stationary position while the index marker is moved to a new position
Slide	The transducer moves across the patient's skin to a new position
Rock	Within same imaging plane the transducer changes orientation either toward or away from the orientation marker

Parasternal Long Axis View

- Usually, the probe is placed in *3rd or 4th ICS* and *the index marker should be towards the right shoulder* of patient **(Figs. 3 and 4)**. Map the heart to get best window for assessment.
- Structures to look for in parasternal long axis (PLAX): From top to bottom
  - Right ventricle (RV) free wall
  - Right ventricular outflow tract (RVOT)
  - Interventricular septum (IVS)
  - Left ventricular outflow tract (LVOT), aortic wall and valves, ascending aorta (AA)
  - LV cavity
  - Mitral valve (MV)
  - Left atrium (LA)
  - LV posterior wall
  - Pericardium
  - Descending thoracic aorta (DTA) and sometime dilated coronary sinus.

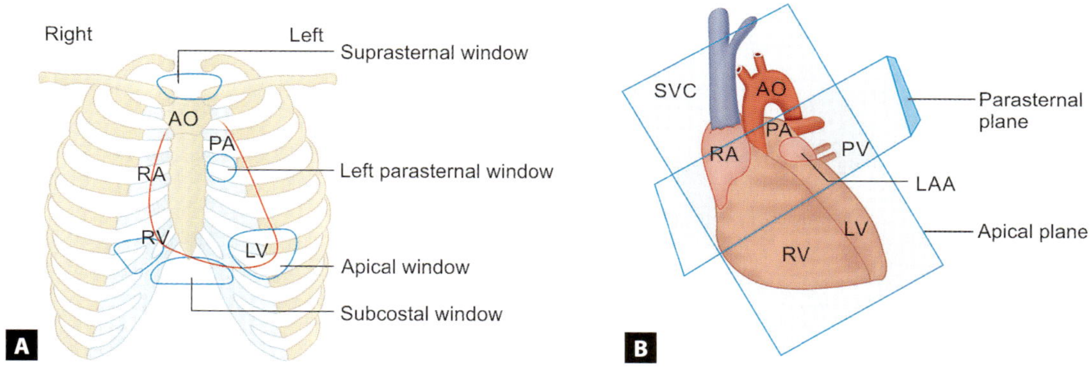

Figs. 2A and B: Schematic diagram showing different echocardiographic window and plane of imaging. (AO: aorta; LAA: left atrial appendage; LV: left ventricle; PA: pulmonary artery; PV: pulmonary vein; RA: right atrium; RV: right ventricle)

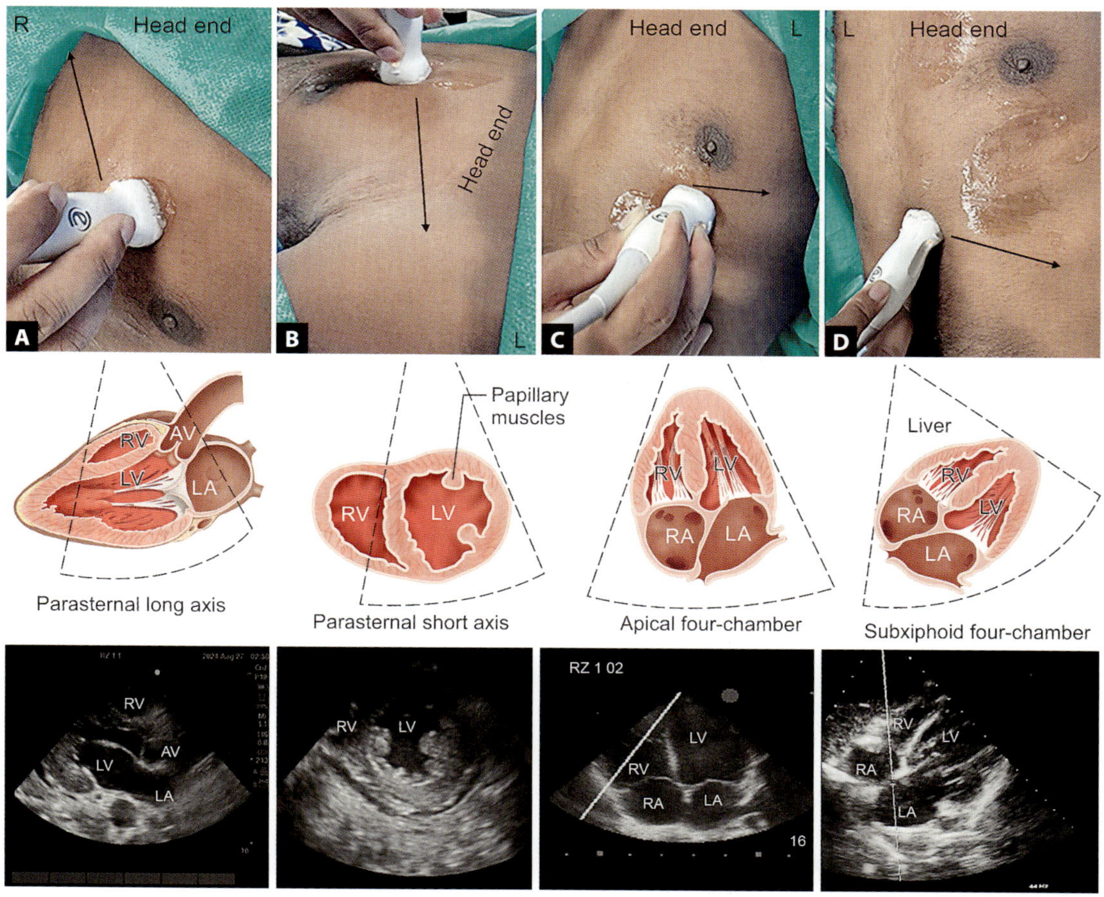

Figs. 3A to D: Probe position and orientation for different echocardiographic windows. (A) Parasternal long axis view; (B) Parasternal short axis; (C) Apical four V chamber; (D) Subxiphoid four-chamber. (AV: aortic valve; LA: left atrium; LV: left ventricle; RV: right ventricle)

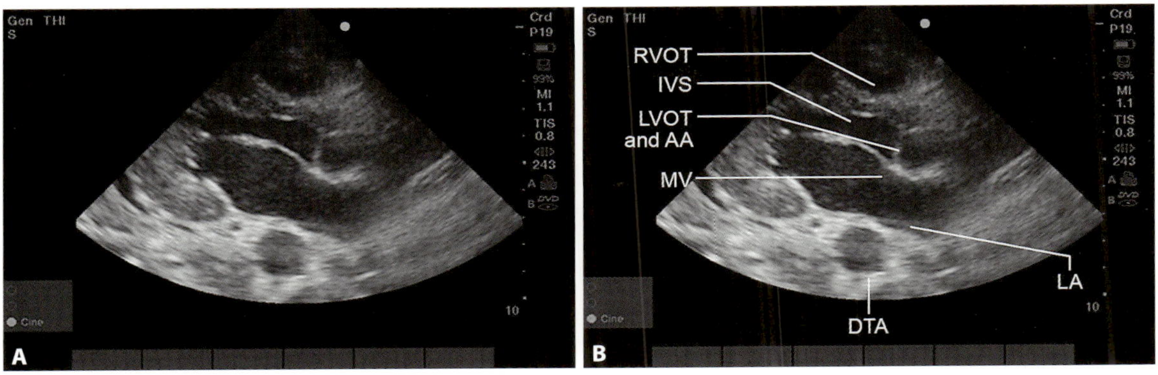

Figs. 4A and B: Parasternal long axis view and structures enumerated. (AA: ascending aorta; DTA: descending thoracic aorta; IVS: interventricular septum; LA: left ventricle; LVOT: left ventricular outflow tract; MV: mitral valve; RVOT: right ventricular outflow tract)

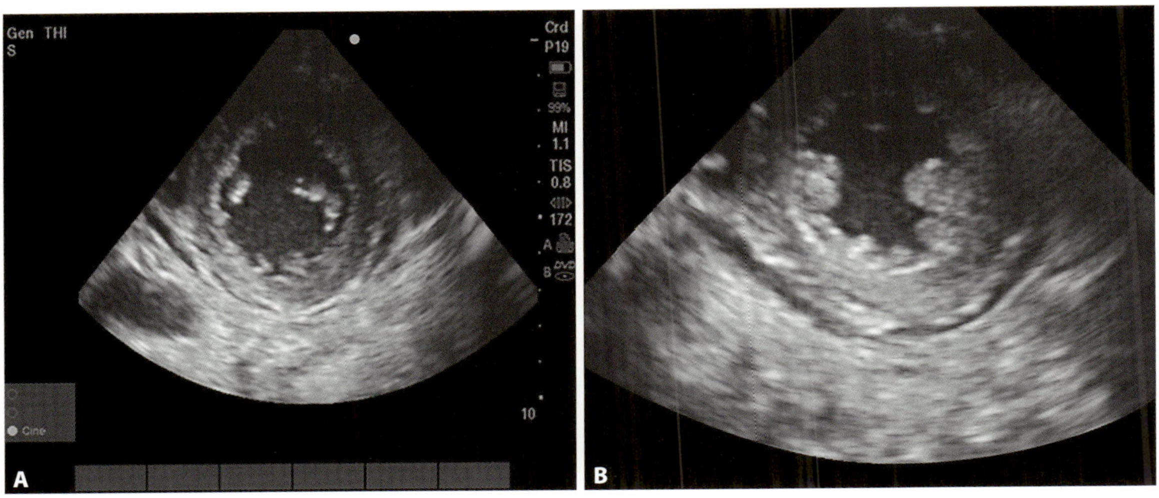

Figs. 5A and B: Parasternal short axis (PSAX) view: (A) Mitral valve level; (B) Mid-papillary level.

Parasternal Short Axis View

- From PLAX view rotate the probe 90° clockwise so that the index marker now points toward left shoulder.
- Slight tilting and rocking of probe give additional four different levels of parasternal short axis (PSAX).
- View all four levels of short axis view of ventricle that includes **(Figs. 3 and 5)**:

1. Apical level (apex)
2. Mid-papillary level (midlevel)
3. MV level
4. Great vessel level

Apical Four-chamber

Find the *point of maximal impulse around 5th ICS*, below the nipple and keep the *pointer at 3 o'clock* map the heart to get good window.

Slight manipulation is required here to obtained window **(Figs. 3 and 6)**. Structures visible here are as follows:

- Left atrium and left ventricle
- Right atrium and RV
- Mitral valve
- Tricuspid valve
- Interatrial septum
- Interventricular septum (inferior wall of septum-inner)
- Lateral wall of left ventricle (outer wall).

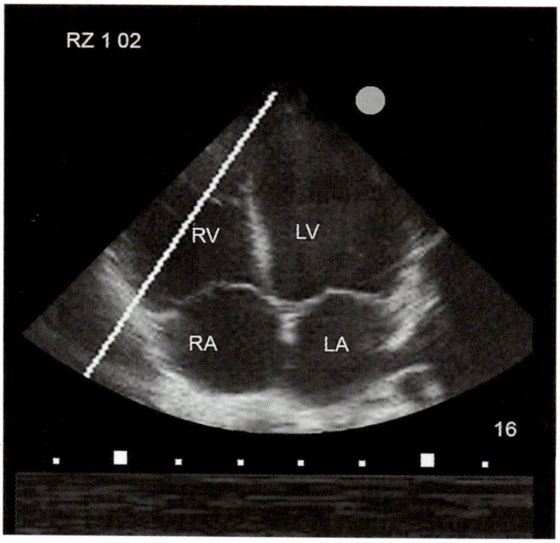

Fig. 6: Apical four-chamber (A4C) view. (LA: left atrium; LV: left ventricle; RA: right atrium; RV: right ventricle)

Apical Five-chamber View

- In the apical view, tilt the tail end probe down toward patient feet without moving clock or anticlockwise
- In addition to structurers seen in four-chamber (4C) view, left ventricular outflow tract, aortic valve, and aorta are visualized **(Figs. 7A and B)**.

Apical Two-chamber View

- From the apical four-chamber (A4C) position, rotate the probe anticlockwise to 12–1 o'clock position to get apical two-chamber (A2C) view
- *Image:* Left atrium and left ventricle **(Figs. 8A and B)**
- Inferior wall and anterior wall of left ventricle seen.

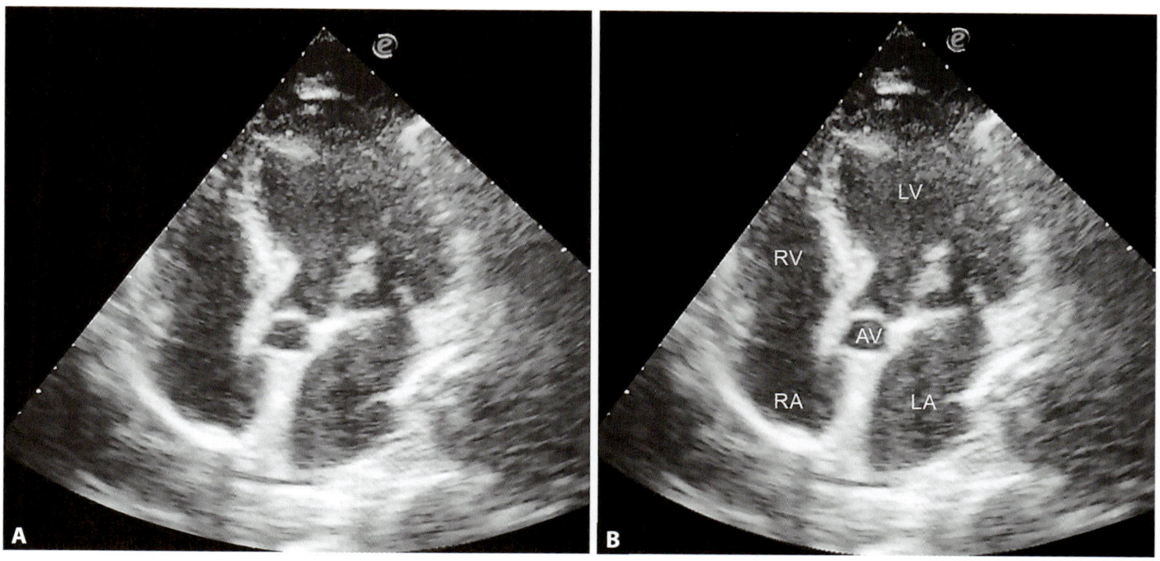

Figs. 7A and B: Apical five-chamber view (left) with structures detailed (right). (AV: aortic valve; LA: left atrium; LV: left ventricle; RA: right atrium; RV: right ventricle)

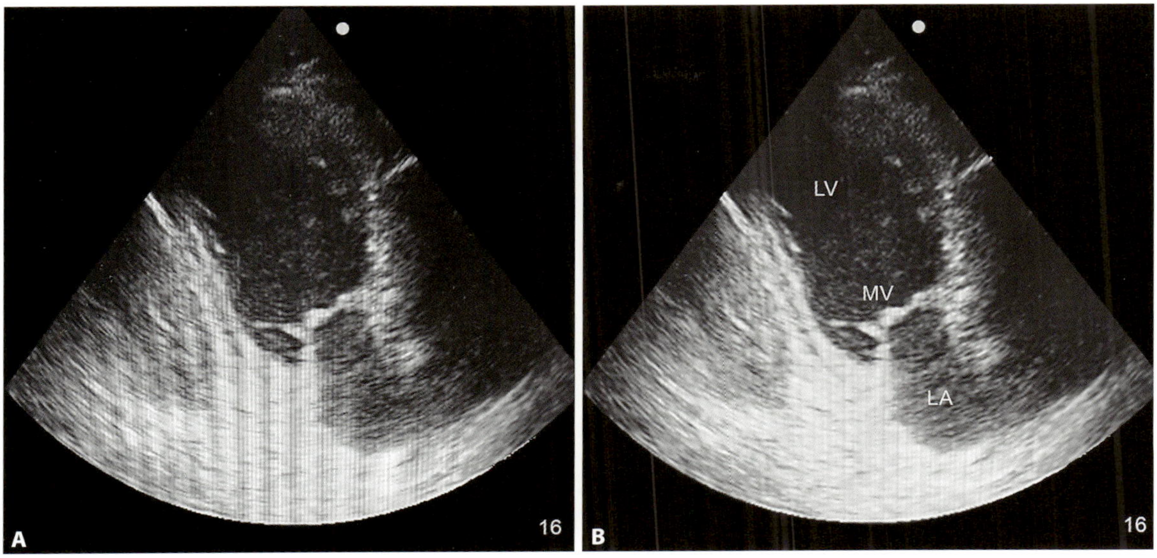

Figs. 8A and B: Apical two-chamber view. (LA: left atrium; LV: left ventricle; MV: mitral valve)

Subcostal View

- Fold the legs and loosen the abdomen of the patient
- Transversely place the probe at epigastrium with index marker facing left side of the patient (similar to A4C view) **(Fig. 3)**.
- Tilt tip of probe down, inter atrial septum and all four chambers are visualized **(Fig. 9)**.
- Tilt probe further down, five-chamber view is visible [like conversion from A4C view to apical five-chamber (A5C) view].
- This view is also used to image inferior vena cava (IVC) by rotating probe anticlockwise and index marker toward head of the patient.
- Marker facing head of patient—IVC seen entering right atrium with hepatic veins draining in IVC.
- This view is very useful in patients on ventilator, unconscious or trauma patients where positioning is difficult.
- Imaging is difficult through this window if abdomen is full.

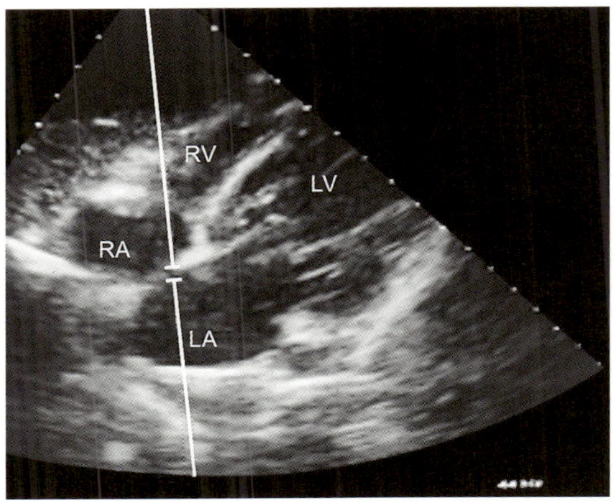

Fig. 9: Subcostal view with structure details. (LA: left atrium; LV: left ventricle; RA: right atrium; RV: right ventricle)

UTILITY OF TWO-DIMENSIONAL ECHOCARDIOGRAPHY IN EMERGENCY

Left Ventricular Function

- Assessment of left ventricular ejection fraction (LVEF)

TABLE 2: Definition of heart failure types.

Types of heart failure	*Criteria*
Heart failure with reduced ejection fraction (HFrEF)	LVEF ≤40%
Heart failure with improved ejection fraction (HFimpEF)	Previous left ventricular ejection fraction (LVEF) <40% and follow-up LVEF >40%
Heart failure with mildly reduced ejection fraction (HFmrEF)	LVEF 41–49% with evidence of increased LV filling pressure
Heart failure with preserved ejection fraction (HFpEF)	LVEF >50% with evidence of increased LV filling pressures

- Formula of LVEF (%) = $\frac{\text{EDV} - \text{ES}}{\text{EDV}} \times 100$

Table 2 shows categorization of heart failure according to LVEF criteria.[1]

- There are several methods to check LVEF out of which Teicholz method and end-point septal separation (EPSS) are useful and easy to learn by beginners.
    - *Eye balling:* It requires practice and skill, most common way to assess LV by emergency physician and intensivist, look at LV wall contractility and thickening during systole, consider multiple view for eye balling.
    - *Teicholz method:*[2] Obtain a good PLAX window with IVS horizontally placed, apex should not be visible. Press M-mode just anterior to tip of MV at IVS. LV diameter from IVS to left ventricular posterior wall (LVPW) during systole and diastole is measured. Most ultrasound machines are enabled with automated calculations. Just pressing for calculations and selecting LVEF leads to automatically generating values of EF and fraction shortening.
    - *Easy way:* Make a good PSAX window, press M-mode, ensure M-mode line transacts ventricle in mid-way as shown below, and take left ventricle diameter in systole and diastole. Machine automatically calculates LVEF **(Fig. 10)**.
    - *Simpsons method:* Obtain A4C view with IVS in perpendicular with apex in the center → You should be able to delineate LV endocardium → trace the LV during diastole and systole → machine automatically calculates ejection fraction
    - *EPSS:*[3] Obtain PLAX window with IVS horizontally placed → press M-mode → place cursor in such a way that it touches tips of MV → M-mode pattern of MV opening during diastole is displayed on screen → calculate the distance between tip of first notch of MV tip to IVS **(Fig. 11)**. Normal value is 7 mm or less, increasing values correlate with worsening ejection fraction.
    - *Mitral annular plane systolic excursion (MAPSE):* Obtain A4C view → visualize the posterior mitral leaflet annulus (viewed laterally) → apply M-mode where posterior mitral leaflet attached to annulus → M-mode trace seen on screen → calculate the maximum height of hump **(Fig. 12)**. Normal value is 12–15 mm, lesser values indicate poor LV systolic function.

Right Heart Assessment

- Difficult due to complex anatomy and shape of RV
- Ways to assess RV function
    - *Tricuspid annular plane systolic excursion (TAPSE):* Obtain A4C view → focus on RV → visualize tricuspid valve annulus → press the M-mode → M-mode trace seen on screen → calculate the maximum height of hump-like MAPSE **(Fig. 13)**. Normal value is 17 mm or more, lesser values indicate poor RV systolic function.

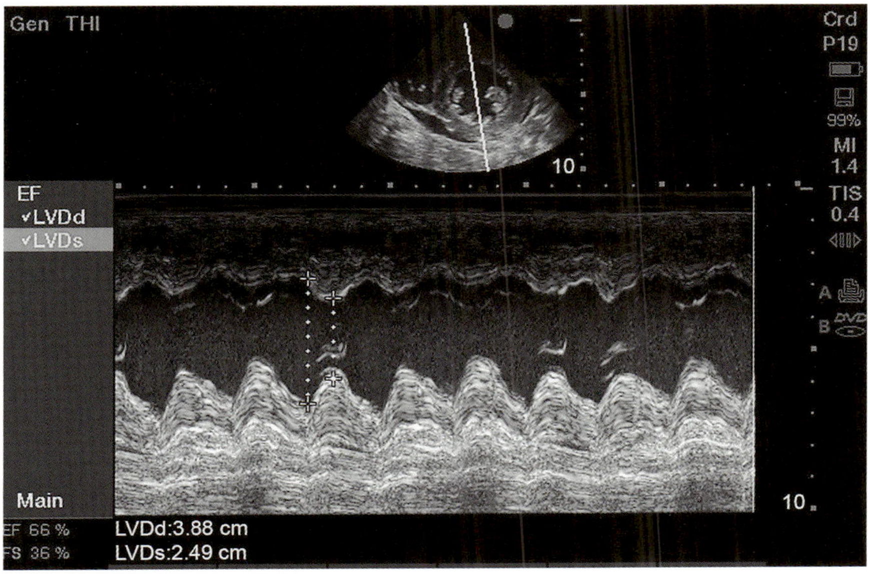

Fig. 10: Teicholz method of assessing left ventricular ejection fraction (LVEF).

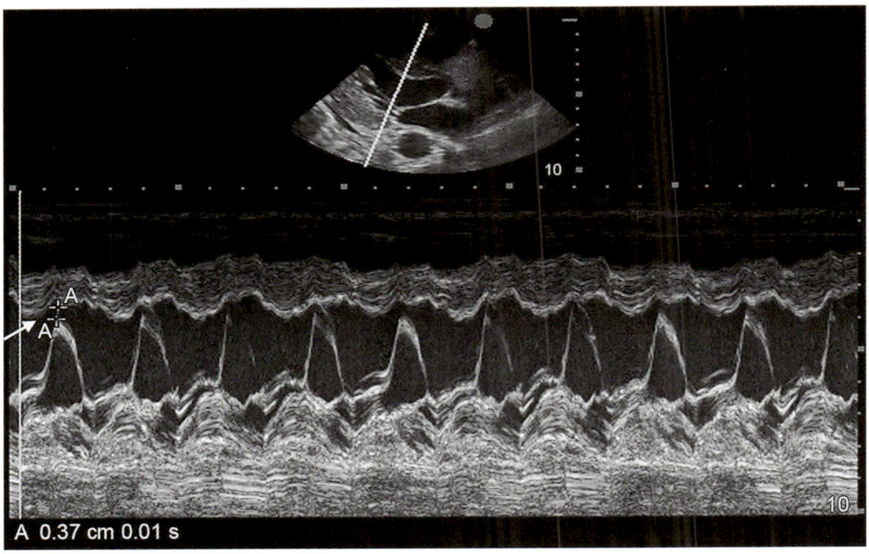

Fig. 11: Measuring end-point septal separation (EPSS).

- *RV S' prime:* It is similar like TAPSE but instead of M-mode apply TDI → measure maximum distance above the baseline **(Fig. 14)**. Normal value is >9.5 cm/second.

Echocardiographic Assessment of Pulmonary Artery Hypertension[4]

Two-dimensional Echo provides a valuable noninvasive method for estimating pulmonary artery pressure.

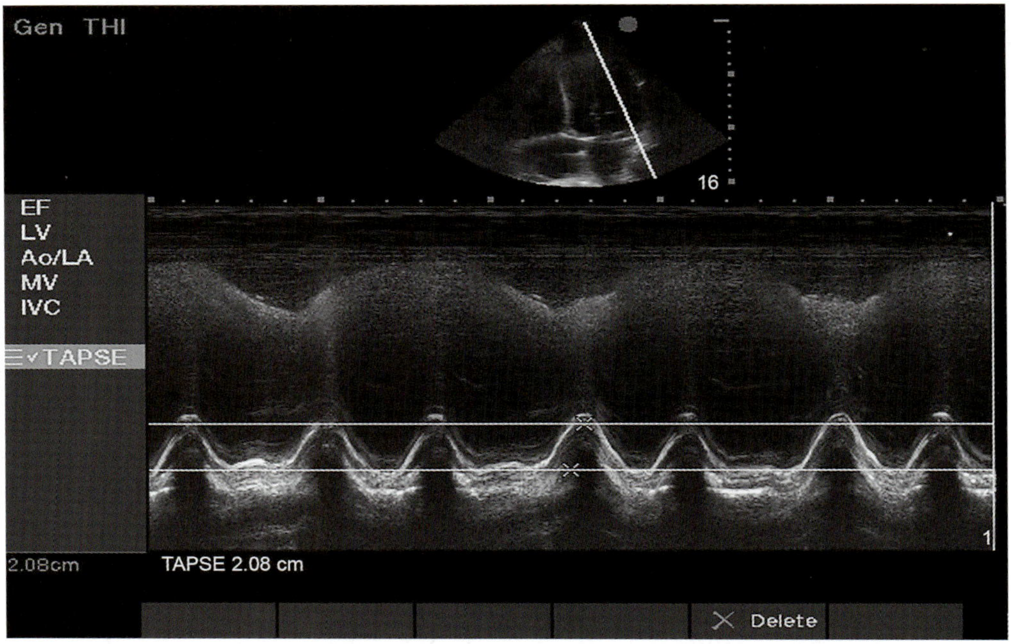

Fig. 12: Mitral annular plane systolic excursion (MAPSE). *Note:* Tricuspid annular plane systolic excursion (TAPSE) function in this machine has been utilized to measure MAPSE.

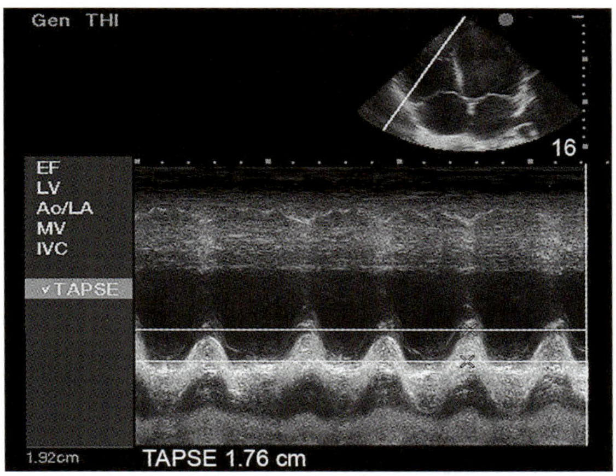

Fig. 13: Assessing tricuspid annular plane systolic excursion (TAPSE).

- *Pulmonary artery systolic pressure (PASP):*
  - This method is used only in presence of tricuspid regurgitation
  - Make a good A4C view, place curser above tricuspid valve → using CW Doppler measure peak velocity of tricuspid regurgitant (TR) flow → machine uses following formula to measure right ventricular systolic pressure (RVSP).

$$\text{RVSP} = 4 \times \text{TR velocity (maximum)} + \text{Right atrial pressure (RAP)}$$

Right atrial pressure is calculated using IVC diameter and collapsibility discussed later in IVC segment. RVSP values help in determining severity of pulmonary hypertension **(Table 3)**.

- *Pulmonary acceleration time (PAT):* Make PSAX view at the level of great vessel, place cursor below pulmonary valve, using CW Doppler, pulmonary flow seen on screen. Measure time to reach peak flow from starting point. PAT can also be used to access severity of pulmonary hypertension **(Table 4)**.
- *60/60 sign for diagnosing acute pulmonary embolism:*[5] Pulmonary acceleration time

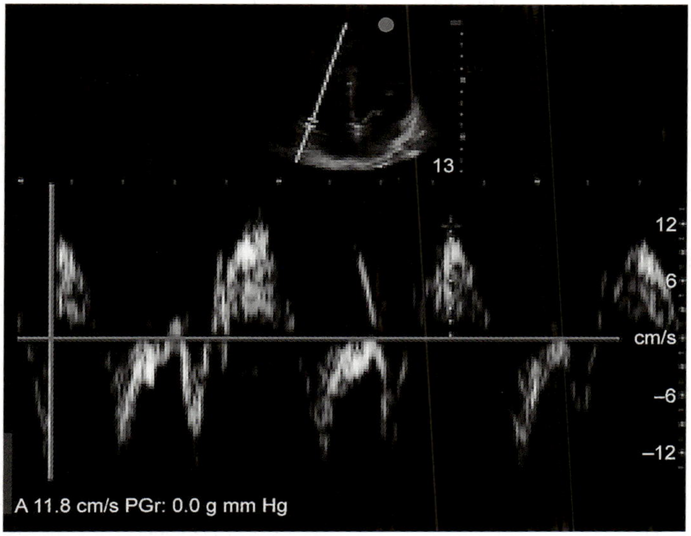

Fig. 14: Application of tissue Doppler imaging (TDI) and obtaining RV S′.

TABLE 3: Severity of pulmonary artery hypertension (PAH) according to RVSP.

RVSP <40 mm Hg (normal)	Severity
40–49	Mild
50–59	Moderate
>60	Severe

(RVSP: right ventricular systolic pressure)

TABLE 4: Severity of pulmonary artery hypertension (PAH) according to pulmonary acceleration time (PAT).

PAT (>120 msec) normal	Severity of pulmonary artery hypertension (PAH)
80–100	Mild
60–80	Moderate
<60	Severe

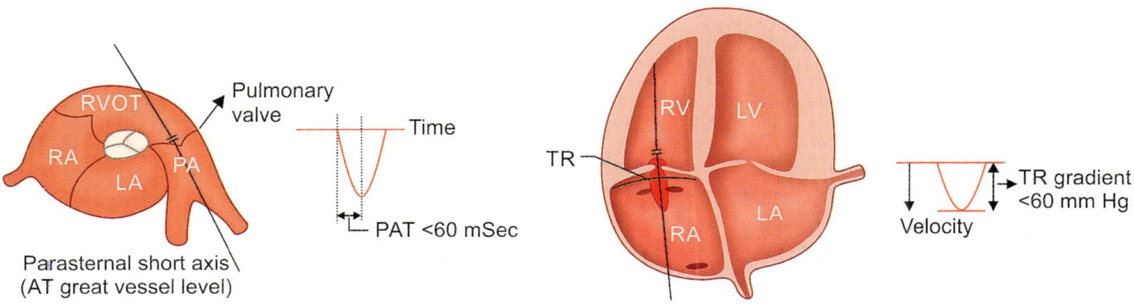

Fig. 15: 60/60 Echo sign of pulmonary thromboembolism. (LA: left atrium; LV: left ventricle; PA: pulmonary artery; PAT: pulmonary acceleration time; TR: tricuspid regurgitation; RVOT: right ventricular outflow tract)

(PAT) <60 mSec and TR pressure gradient <60 mm Hg (but >30 mm Hg): Indirect indicator of pulmonary thromboembolism **(Fig. 15)**.

Additional Echo findings of pulmonary artery hypertension (PAH) are dilated RA, RV, pulmonary artery, and RV hypertrophy.

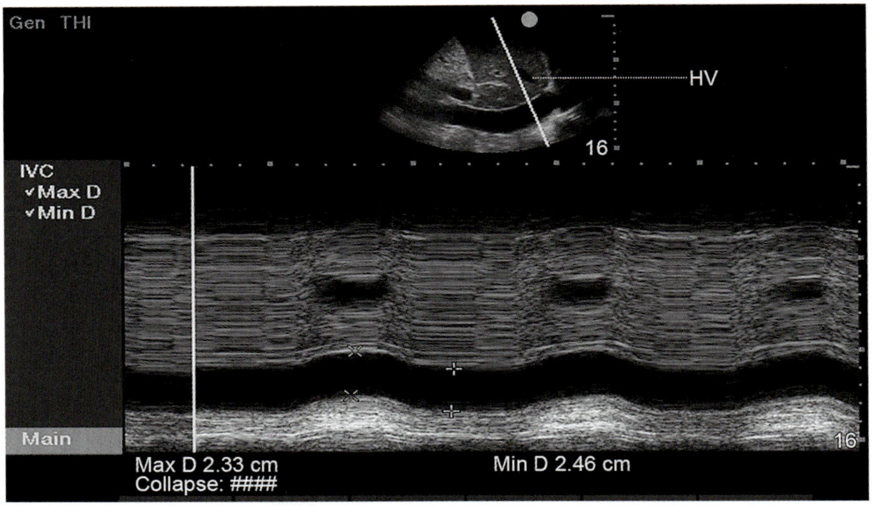

Fig. 16: Inferior vena cava (IVC) measurement in M-mode showing respiratory variations.

Inferior Vena Cava Measurement

- *IVC* measurement can help in determining status of RAP and intravascular volume status **(Fig. 16)**.
- *IVC is usually measured 1-2 cm distal to hepatic vein.*
- *Normal size of IVC is <17 mm.*
- Collapsibility measured by putting M-mode at 1–2 cm distal to hepatic vein.[6]

$$\text{Collapsibility index} = \frac{\text{IVC maximum} - \text{IVC minimum}}{(\text{IVC maximum})} \times 100$$

- IVC diameter and collapsibility gives an estimate of the RAP **(Table 5)**.

TABLE 5: Mean RAP assessment depending on IVC diameter and collapsibility.

IVC diameter	*IVC collapse*	*Mean RAP (mm Hg)*
<1.5 cm	Total collapse (100%)	0–5
1.5–2.5	>50%	6–10
1.5–2.5	<50%	11–15
>2.5	<50%	16–20
>2.5	0% no collapsibility	>20

(IVC: inferior vena cava; RAP: right atrial pressure)

Aortic Diameter

Screening aortic diameter measurement at two places is must to rule out aortic aneurysm **(Figs. 17A and B)**.

1. Ascending aortic diameter at sinotubular junction (22–36 mm normal value) >40 mm (suggestive of aortic aneurism).
   It is measured by making PLAX window on screen.
2. Abdominal aortic diameter (approximately 20 mm normal value) >30 mm (suggestive of abdominal aortic aneurysm).

Seen through subcostal window placing transducer index marker toward head.

Pericardial Effusion

- Subcostal view is often the easiest and most reliable to see pericardial effusion and its measurement **(Fig. 18)**.

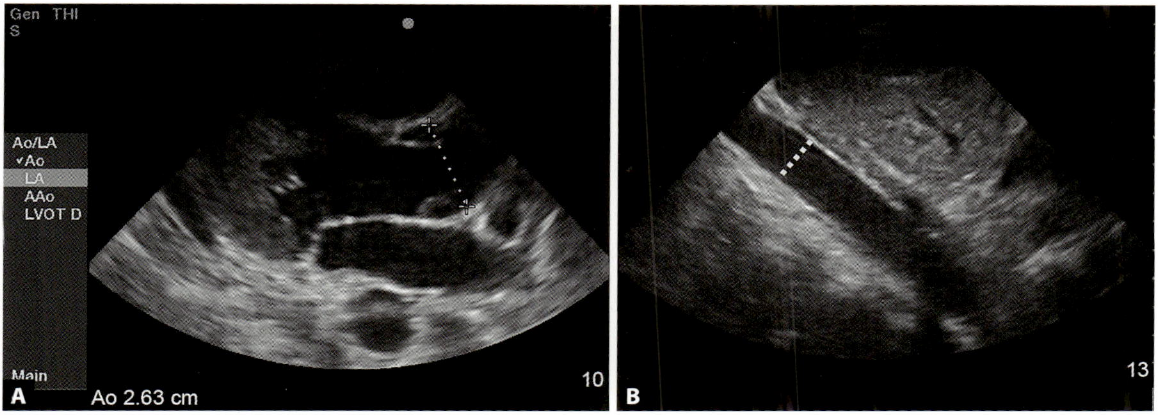

Figs. 17A and B: *Assessment of aorta:* (A) Parasternal long axis (PLAX) view; (B) Abdominal aorta.

TABLE 6: Severity of pericardial effusion.

Pericardial effusion severity	*Measurement*
Mild	10 mm (50–100 mL)
Moderate	10–20 mm (100–500 mL)
Severe	>20 mm (>500 mL)

- Pericardial effusion is measured by size of largest width of effusion at the end of diastole **(Table 6)**.
- Early RV diastolic collapse and late RA systolic collapse, dilated IVC, and reduced collapsibility are features of cardiac tamponade on 2D echocardiography.

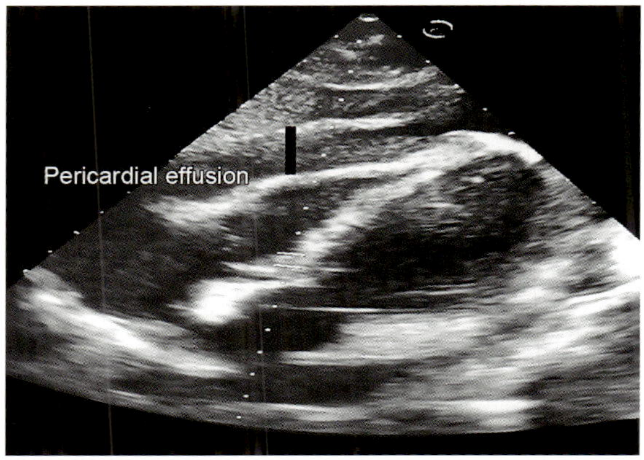

Fig. 18: Assessment of pericardial effusion.

CONCLUSION

Emergency physicians are usually first point of contact of sick patients requiring hospital admission. Being aware of basics of echocardiography enables physicians to diagnose cardiac emergencies and other life-threatening conditions early such as acute heart failure, cardiac tamponade, pulmonary embolism, cardiogenic shock, hypovolemia of patient that help in appropriate fluid resuscitation, infective endocarditis as a cause of sepsis, valve function, and cardiogenic pulmonary edema. Early diagnosis leads to early effective management and hence reduced morbidity and mortality.

REFERENCES

1. Shams P, Goyal A, Makaryus AN. Left Ventricular Ejection Fraction. In: StatPearls [Internet]. Treasure Island (FL): StatPearls Publishing; 2025.
2. Arora G, Morss AM, Piazza G, Ryan JW, Dinwoodey DL, Rofsky NM, et al. Differences in left ventricular ejection fraction using teichholz formula and volumetric methods by CMR: implications for patient stratification and selection of therapy. J Cardiovasc Magn Reson. 2010;12(Suppl 1):P202.

3. Joshi P, Borde D, Asegaonkar B, Daunde V, Joshi S, Jaspara A. Utility of E point septal separation as screening tool for left ventricular ejection fraction in perioperative settings by anesthetists. Ann Card Anaesth. 2022;25(3):304-10.
4. Augustine DX, Coates-Bradshaw LD, Willis J, Harkness A, Ring L, Grapsa J, et al. Echocardiographic assessment of pulmonary hypertension: a guideline protocol from the British Society of Echocardiography. Echo Res Pract. 2018;5(3):G11-G24.
5. Kurzyna M, Torbicki A, Pruszczyk P, Burakowska B, Fijałkowska A, Kober J, et al. Disturbed right ventricular ejection pattern as a new Doppler echocardiographic sign of acute pulmonary embolism. Am J Cardiol. 2002;90(5):507-11.
6. Kaptein MJ, Kaptein EM. Inferior Vena Cava Collapsibility Index: Clinical Validation and Application for Assessment of Relative Intravascular Volume. Adv Chronic Kidney Dis. 2021;28(3):218-26.

CHAPTER 6

Abdominal Ultrasound

Chetna Shamshery, Ashish Kumar Kannaujia

WHAT YOU WILL LEARN IN THIS CHAPTER?

A. Basic anatomy and surface marking for abdominal ultrasound

B. Indications

C. Equipment setup and step-by-step approach to acute abdomen scan

INTRODUCTION

Acute abdomen is a condition which requires immediate medical attention and accounts for the third most frequent complain with which patients report in emergency department (ED) to the physicians.[1] Acute pain may be diffuse or localized with most common causes being cholecystitis, appendicitis, bowel obstruction, aneurysm, trauma, and stones in kidney or gallbladder. A few conditions such as hemorrhage, obstruction, bleed, or perforation may require immediate surgical interventions.[2,3] Despite the fact that time is a critical factor in an emergency setting, only 2–3% physicians use bedside ultrasound (USG) as a diagnostic aid in their approach to manage acute emergencies. This chapter explores the applications, and interpretation of abdominal USG in ED, its diagnostic value, limitations, and specific protocols used in critical scenarios.

WHY ABDOMINAL SONOGRAPHY IN EMERGECNY?

- Abdominal USG is a dynamic and focused scan performed by a nonradiologists at the bedside, which can aid in spotting the diagnosis and management in over 50% of the cases of acute abdomen. It should be preceded by history taking and clinical examination.
- Bedside USG is a fast, noninvasive, and effective means to diagnose wide range of conditions, triaging patient management and ensuring rapid decision-making.[4]
- Portability, availability, repeatability, and lack of radiation exposure has made USG the first and most feasible imaging modality during hours of need especially in pregnant or women of reproductive age groups.
- Cochrane review supports the use of USG for bedside point of care assessment for thoracoabdominal trauma in adult population but advises confirmation by computed tomography (CT) for acute abdominal emergencies.[5]
- This has also been recommended in order to avoid overexposure and misuse of CT as an imaging modality for relatively nontraumatic less severe abdominal conditions, as routine scan of abdomen may lead to unnecessary findings which in majority of cases may not require a significant medical intervention.[1]

ANATOMY AND SURFACE MARKING

- To understand the basic structural anatomy for emergencies, the abdomen is either divided into four quadrants or nine segments by two vertical lines passing from midclavicular points on either side and two horizontal lines, one subcostal drawn through inferior aspect of lowest costal cartilage and second through the highest point of iliac crest **(Fig. 1)**.

- The underlying visceral anatomy and the cause for acute abdomen accordingly has been tabulated in **Table 1**.
- It is to be emphasized that despite pain being referred to any one particular segment, it is necessary to scan the whole of abdomen in order to avoid missing any significant findings.[6]

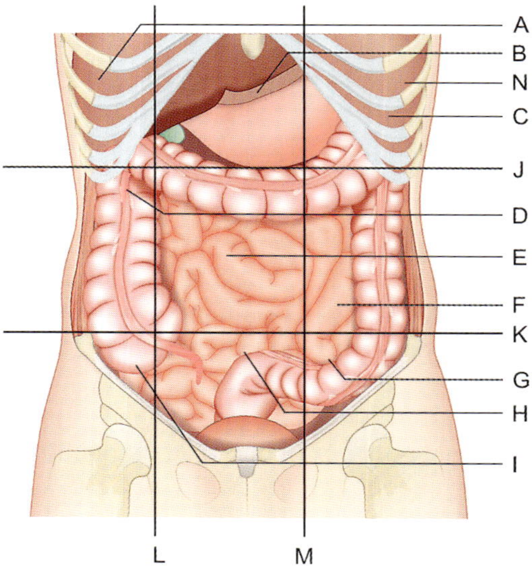

Fig. 1: Division of abdomen into nine segments demonstrating the underlying viscera.

INDICATIONS FOR ABDOMINAL ULTRASOUND IN EMERGENCY[7]

- *Trauma:* Focused Assessment with Sonography for Trauma (FAST) protocol helps to detect abdominal bleed even if minimal up to 60 mL in patients subjected to physical trauma, especially when the collection is hidden in the hepatorenal pouch, splenorenal recess, pelvic girdle, and pericardial space.
- *Perforation:* Identification of intraperitoneal free fluid (IPF) and air can be diagnosed with a minimum of 10 mL collection. Although this finding is to be confirmed using contrast CT.
- *Vascular scan:* Inferior vena cava scan to see the fluid status of patients in emergency and assess the dynamic fluid response.
- Aortic aneurysm or dissection is diagnosed with high sensitivity and specificity.
- Acute abdomen due to inflammation or colicky pain due to obstruction of appendix, gallbladder, bowel, and kidney. Acute appendicitis has high specificity (96%) with USG.
- *Assessment of liver and spleen:* Evaluation for size, texture, and obvious pathology of liver and spleen.
- *Bladder evaluation:* Measurement of postvoid residual volume, detection of bladder distention, or urinary retention.

TABLE 1: Segmental division with underlying visceral anatomy and etiology of acute abdomen.

Surface marking	*Area scanned*	*Viscera underlying*	*Acute abdomen etiology*
A	Right hypochondrium	Liver	Traumatic bleed/hepatitis
		Right kidney	Stones/pyelonephritis/hydronephrosis
		Small and large intestine	Obstruction/intussusception/perforation
		Gallbladder	Cholecystitis/gallstones/cholangitis
B	Epigastrium	Liver	Traumatic bleed/hepatitis
		Pancreas	Pancreatitis
		Stomach	Ulcer/perforation

Contd...

Contd...

Surface marking	***Area scanned***	***Viscera underlying***	***Acute abdomen etiology***
		Duodenum	Perforation
		Aorta	Aneurysm/dissection
C	Left hypo-chondrium	Liver	Traumatic bleed/hepatitis
		Left kidney	Colic due to stones/pyelonephritis
		Stomach	Ulcer/perforation
		Spleen	Traumatic bleed/splenomegaly
		Small and large intestine	Obstruction/intussusception/perforation
D	Right lumbar	Ascending colon	Obstruction/intussusception/perforation
		Small intestine	
		Right kidney	Stones/hydronephrosis/pyelonephritis
E	Umbilical	Duodenum	Perforation
		Transverse colon	Obstruction/intussusception/perforation
		Small intestine	
		Abdominal aorta and internal iliac artery	Aneurysm/dissection
F	Left lumbar	Descending colon	Obstruction/intussusception/perforation/colitis/diverticulitis
		Small intestine	
		Left kidney	Colic due to stones/hydronephrosis
G	Right iliac	Appendix	Appendicitis
		Cecum	Obstruction/intussusception/perforation/hernia
		Ascending colon	
		Small intestine	
		Ovary	Torsion/cyst
H	Hypo-gastrium	Bladder	Urinary retention/urinary tract infection
		Sigmoid colon	Obstruction/intussusception/perforation
		Small intestine	
		Reproductive organs	Ectopic pregnancy/ovarian cyst/testicular torsion
I	Left iliac	Sigmoid colon	Diverticulitis/obstruction/intussusception/perforation/hernia
		Descending colon	
		Small intestine	
		Ovary	Torsion/cyst
J	Upper horizontal line passing from lowest costal cartilages		
K	Lower horizontal line passing from the highest point of iliac crest		
L	First vertical line from right mid clavicular point		
M	Second vertical line from left mid clavicular point		
N	Diaphragm lining		

- USG is diagnostic modality of choice for pregnancy-related emergencies especially life-threatening ectopic pregnancy.
- Diagnosis and drainage of ascites under real-time USG can be reliably performed when the patient lies in left or right lateral decubitus. In cases of massive ascites leading to breathlessness, it gives immediate relief.

EQUIPMENT SETUP AND PROBE SELECTION

- *Curvilinear (low frequency) transducer (2–5 MHz):* This is the most common probe used for abdominal scanning. It has deeper penetration but relatively poorer resolution.
- *Phased array (low frequency) transducer:* While typically used for cardiac imaging, it can also be used in the FAST examination to detect free fluid in trauma, especially in pericardial pockets or to detect fluid status of the patient for inferior vena cava scan.
- *Linear (high frequency) transducer (6–13 MHz):* It is mainly to detect air in peritoneum due to perforation.

STEPS OF ABDOMINAL POINT-OF-CARE ULTRASOUND[8]

1. *Focused assessment with sonography for trauma*
   - *Indications:* In patients subjected to one or other form of physical trauma, to look for collection of blood.
   - *Probe positioning and possible findings* **(Figs. 2A to L)**:
     - *Subxiphoid:* Place the curvilinear/ phased array probe just below the xiphoid process with some cranial and leftward tilt to see blood in pericardial or pleural space **(Figs. 2A, 2E, and 2I)**.
     - *Morrison's pouch (right upper quadrant):* Place the curvilinear probe in right subcostal region and slide

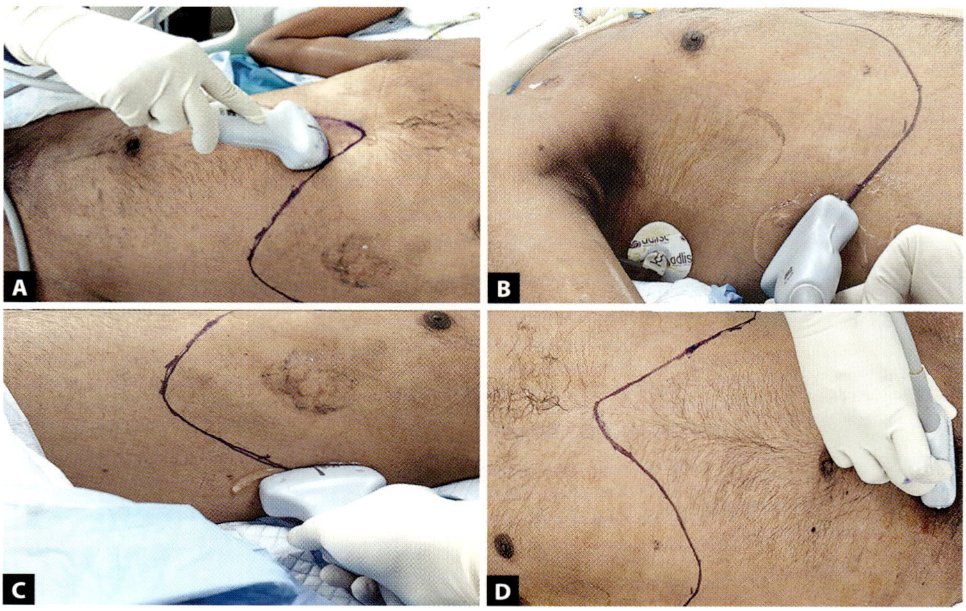

Figs. 2A to D

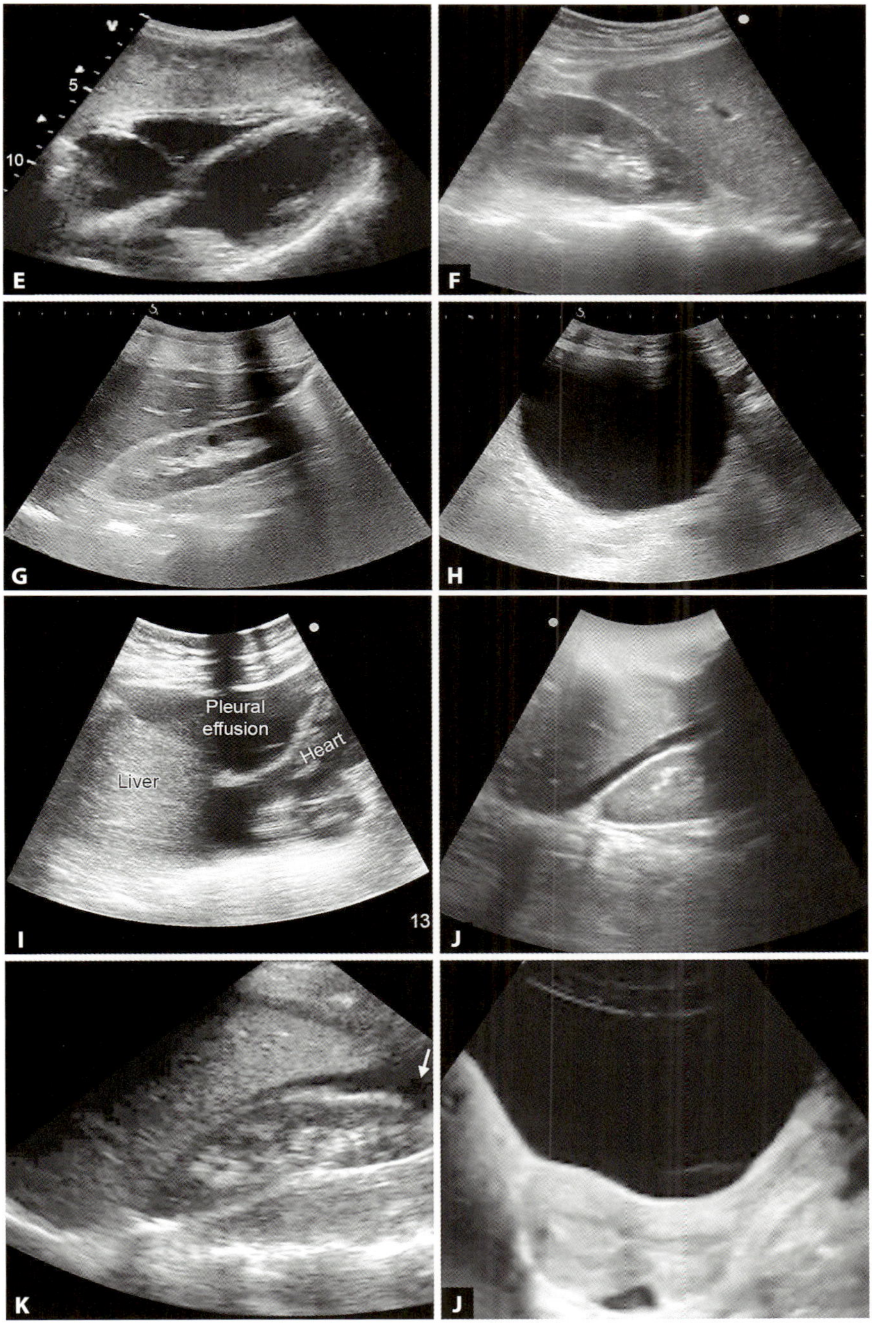

Figs. 2E to L

Figs. 2A to L: (A to D) Probe positioning; (E to H) Normal sonographic images in different positions; (I) Subxiphoid view with pleural effusion; (J) Fluid in hepatorenal space, Focused Assessment with Sonography in Trauma (FAST) positive; (K) Fluid in splenorenal space, FAST positive; (L) Fluid in pelvic area.

it obliquely or longitudinally from anterior to mid axillary line to visualize collection in the hepatorenal space **(Figs. 2B, 2F, and 2J).**
    - *Splenorenal space (left upper quadrant):* Place the curvilinear probe in left subcostal region and slide it obliquely or longitudinally from anterior to midaxillary line to visualize collection in the splenorenal space **(Figs. 2C, 2G, and 2K)**.
    - *Pelvic:* Place the curvilinear probe below the umbilicus and move up to pubic symphysis, to visualize blood behind the urinary bladder in the rectouterine or rectovesical pouch **(Figs. 2D, 2H, and 2L)**.
    - In more skilled hands, the kidney, liver, or spleen laceration can also be appreciated.
- *Key findings:* Echogenicity may help to identify if collection is fresh blood or ascitic fluid which appears anechoic or clotted blood which appears gray or isoechoic with the adjacent structures.

2. *Intraperitoneal scan for free air and fluid*
    - *Indications:* Bleed/perforation/ascites due to inflammation of intestine, gastric ulcer, trauma, malignancy, ruptured ectopic pregnancy, biliary leak, and urinary leak.
    - *Probe positioning:* Linear high-frequency probe, transverse position starting from epigastrium **(Fig. 3A)**.
    - *Technique:* Scan midline region of abdomen first, starting from the epigastrium, umbilical, and hypogastrium, followed by right hypochondrium and the rest of abdomen to observe collection of air in the peritoneum. Position of the patient remains supine with 30° head lift. Patient can also be tilted toward any one side to make fluid collection dependent. **Figure 3B** shows a normal abdominal scan.
    - *Key findings:* Presence of intraperitoneal free fluid or air with reverberations/comet tail appearance at air mucosa interface along with associated decreased intestinal motility or ileus and thickened bowel loops **(Fig. 3C)**.[9,10]
    - Position of the gas and its correlation with the site of perforation requires advanced learning skills and is not being dealt in this chapter.

3. *Obstruction of bowel/appendix*
    - *Indications:* Acute abdomen with or without abdominal distention
    - *Probe positioning:*
        - *For appendix:* Place linear probe between umbilicus and anterior superior iliac spine (ASIS) which is the McBurney's point **(Fig. 4A)**.

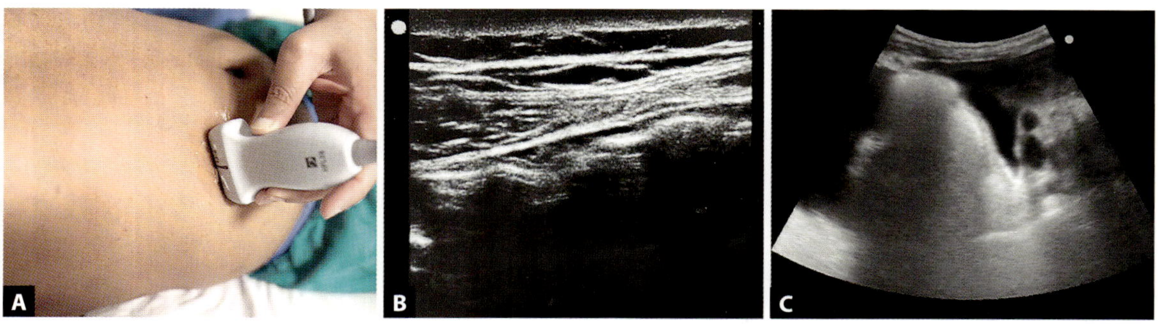

Figs. 3A to C: (A) Ultrasound (USG) probe placement in right hypochondrium with patient in lateral tilt; (B) USG abdomen showing peritoneum and intestinal shadow without ascites; (C) Showing intraperitoneal free fluid with floating bowel loops.

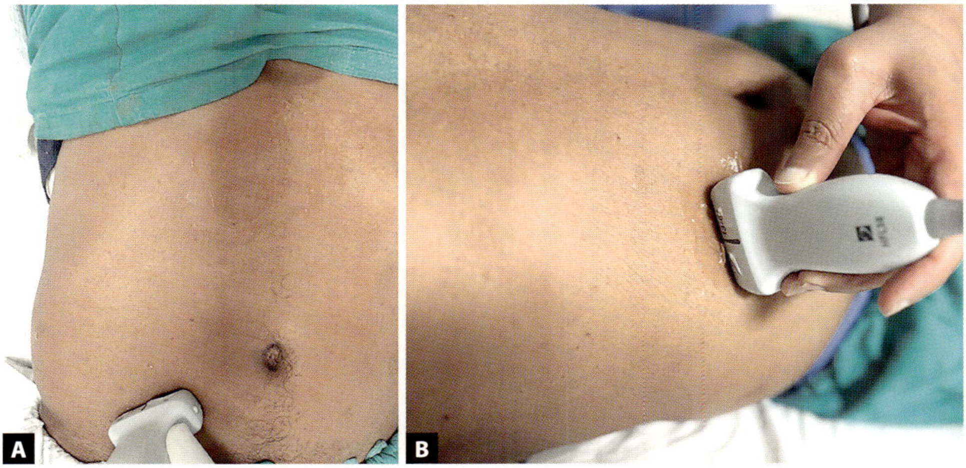

Figs. 4A and B: (A) Probe positioning for appendix scan; (B) Probe positioning for bowel scan.

- For obstructed bowel, scanning needs to be done over whole abdomen **(Fig. 4B)**.
- *Technique:* Appendix will not be seen if it is not inflamed as it is retrocecal most of the times. Upon inflammation, it will be seen as a noncompressible tubular structure known as "target sign" with measurement of >6 mm. Obstructed bowel would be seen as dilated loops with sluggish or absent bowel peristalsis and thickening of bowel walls.

4. *Liver, gallbladder, and evaluation*[11,12]
   - *Indications:* Hepatomegaly, any mass or lesion, cholecystitis, cholelithiasis, and appendicitis
   - *Probe positioning for liver and gallbladder:* Place the curvilinear probe in the right upper quadrant or the mid axillary space between 9th and 11th intercostal space with the probe indicator facing toward the patient's head (longitudinal) or right (transverse) **(Figs. 5A and B)**.
   - *Technique:* Scan the liver for size, echogenicity [should be isoechoic **(Fig. 5C)**, hypo- or hyperechoic may be signs of hepatitis or cirrhosis respectively] and masses. Probe placed longitudinally in the subcostal area may show "Mickey Mouse sign" which shows portal vein as head and common bile duct (CBD) and hepatic artery as ears in short axis view **(Fig. 5E)**. Evaluate the gallbladder for the presence of stones or signs of cholecystitis (thickened walls and pericholecystic fluid).
   - *Key findings:* Liver normal size of <16 cm **(Fig. 5D)**, gallstones, sludge, or evidence of acute cholecystitis (wall thickening >3 mm, distention >4 cm, or pericholecystic fluid) **(Figs. 5F to H)**.
5. *Spleen evaluation*[12,13]
   - *Probe positioning:* Place the curvilinear probe in the left upper quadrant mid- or posterior axillary space, in 7th to 9th intercostal space aligning it to visualize the spleen under the ribs **(Fig. 6A)**.
   - *Technique:* Scan the spleen for size, shape, and any masses. Normal length is <12 cm; no free fluid **(Fig. 6B)**. Ensure to look for free fluid in the perisplenic space, especially in trauma cases.

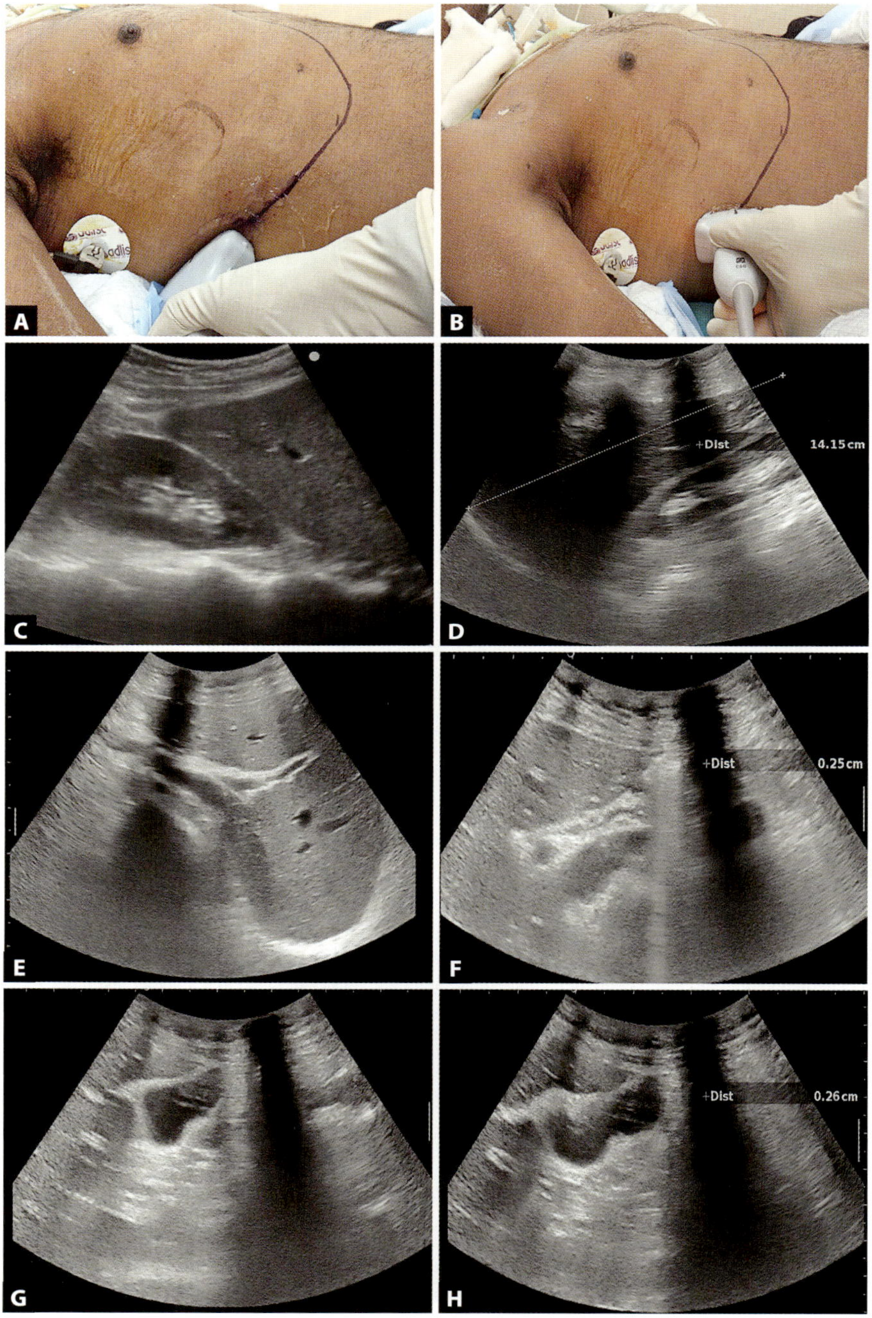

Figs. 5A to H: (A and B) Probe in midaxillary space with probe oblique (A) and longitudinal (B) placement; (C) Hepatorenal space with posterior spine shadows; (D) Measuring liver size from highest point of liver subdiaphragmatically; (E) Ultrasound (USG) probe positioned in oblique plane in subcostal shows liver with portal vein (thick walled); (F) Common bile duct; (G) Gallbladder; (H) Gallbladder with wall measurements for cholecystitis.

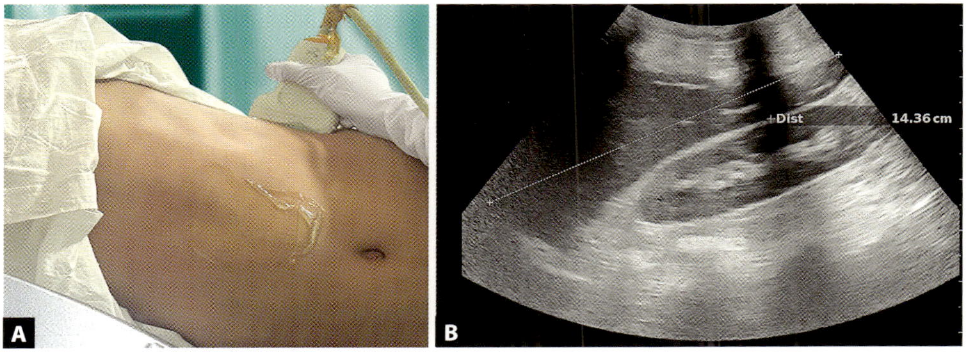

Figs. 6A and B: *Scan for spleen evaluation:* (A) Probe positioning; (B) Splenic view with left kidney.

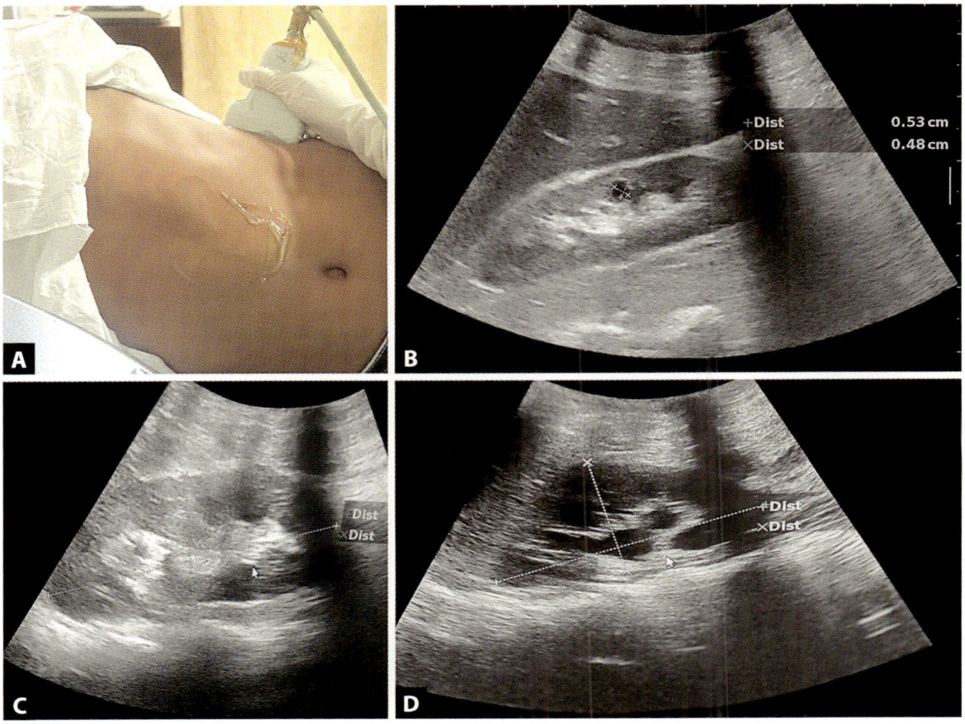

Figs. 7A to D: Ultrasound (USG) evaluation for kidney; (A) Probe positioning; (B) USG picture of left kidney with spleen; (C) Renal stones; (D) Hydronephrosis.

- *Key findings:* Splenomegaly (>12 cm), masses, or free fluid around the spleen.

6. *Kidney evaluation*[14]
   - *Probe positioning:* Place the probe in the posterior axillary line, with the indicator pointing upward to scan the kidney longitudinally **(Fig. 7A)**.
   - *Technique:* Scan both kidneys for size and normal cortical thickness **(Fig. 7B)**.
   - *Key findings:* Look for cystic lesion any mass, stones **(Fig. 7C)** or dilated renal pelvis and calyces which are signs of hydronephrosis **(Fig. 7D)**.

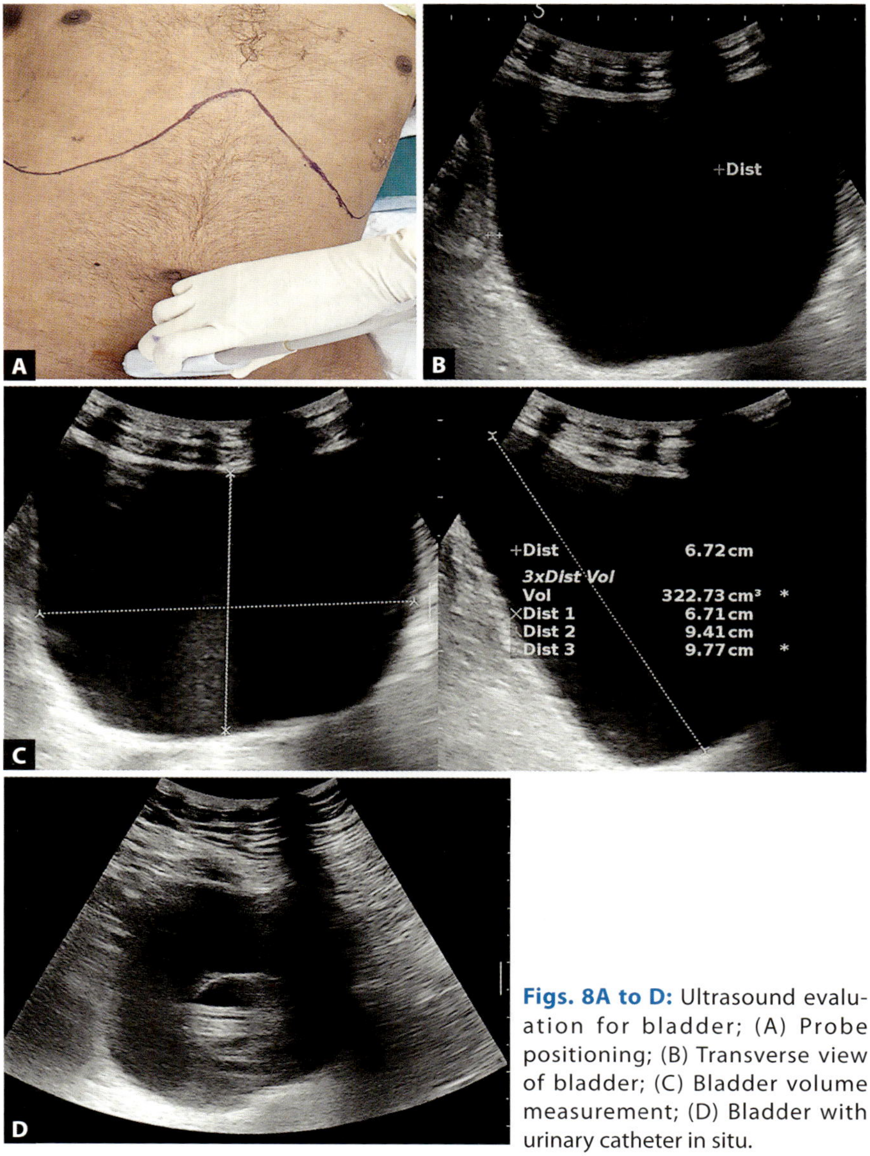

Figs. 8A to D: Ultrasound evaluation for bladder; (A) Probe positioning; (B) Transverse view of bladder; (C) Bladder volume measurement; (D) Bladder with urinary catheter in situ.

7. *Bladder evaluation*[15]
   - *Probe positioning:* Place the linear/curvilinear probe in the suprapubic region in transverse **(Fig. 8A)** as well as longitudinal position.
   - *Technique:* Evaluate the bladder's shape and volume **(Fig. 8B)**. In cases of suspected urinary retention, measure the bladder dimensions to calculate the volume **(Fig. 8C)**.
   - *Key findings:* Bladder with urinary catheter in situ **(Fig. 8D)** distention or residual volume >100 mL after voiding suggests urinary retention.

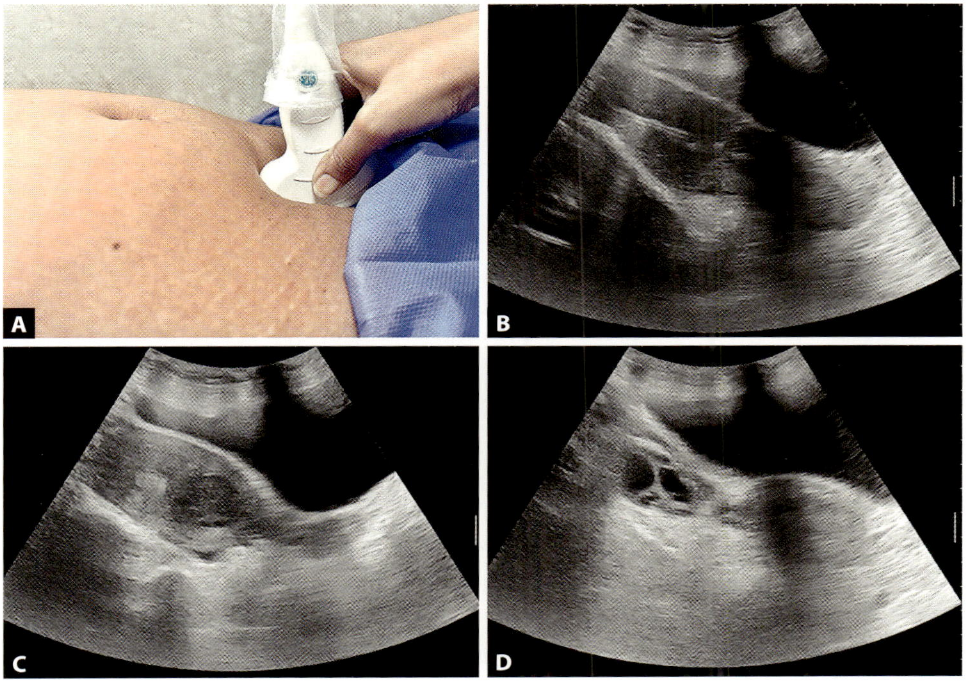

Figs. 9A to D: (A) Longitudinal probe placement for uterine scan; (B) Copper-T in situ; (C) Uterine cavity with fibroid; (D) Showing ovarian cyst.

8. *Uterine scan*[16]
   - *Probe positioning:* Place the curvilinear probe in the suprapubic region in transverse as well as longitudinal position **(Fig. 9A)**.
   - *Technique:* Evaluate the uterine cavity for fetus, any mass, or any other abnormal findings.
   - *Key findings:* Document evidence of ectopic pregnancy during severe abdominal pain and shock with presence of free fluid in peritoneum, absence of intrauterine fetus, thickened echogenic endometrium, and high β-human chorionic gonadotropin (β-hCG) levels (positive pregnancy test). **Figures 9B to D** show various other possible findings in uterine scan.
9. *Costophrenic angles*[17]
   - *Probe positioning:* Place the probe obliquely in the posterior midaxillary space **(Fig. 10A)**.
   - *Technique:* Evaluate both sides and ask the patient to breathe deeply and see the diaphragmatic movements **(Fig. 10B)**, along with any consolidation or collection in the costophrenic angle **(Fig. 10C)**.
   - *Key findings:* Rule out any collection or basal atelectasis.
10. *Ultrasound-guided abdominal interventions in emergency*[18]
   - *Indications:* Therapeutic or diagnostic tap, paracentesis.
   - *Probe:* Linear/curvilinear probe with patient in right or left lateral tilt position.
   - *Technique:* Scan whole abdomen to look for intraperitoneal free fluid with left or right lateral tilt to make the fluid accumulate in a dependent area **(Figs. 11A and B)**. Insert tapping needle under USG guidance and aspirate the fluid **(Fig. 11C)**.

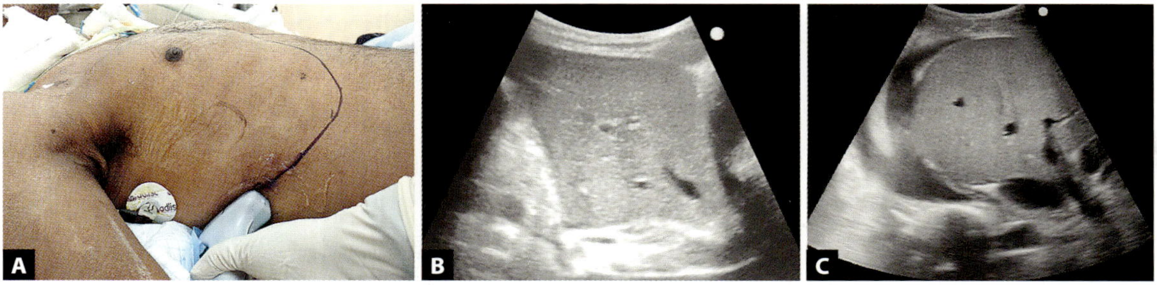

Figs. 10A to C: (A) Oblique probe positioning for costophrenic angle scan; (B) Normal costophrenic window; (C) Pleural effusion in ultrasound.

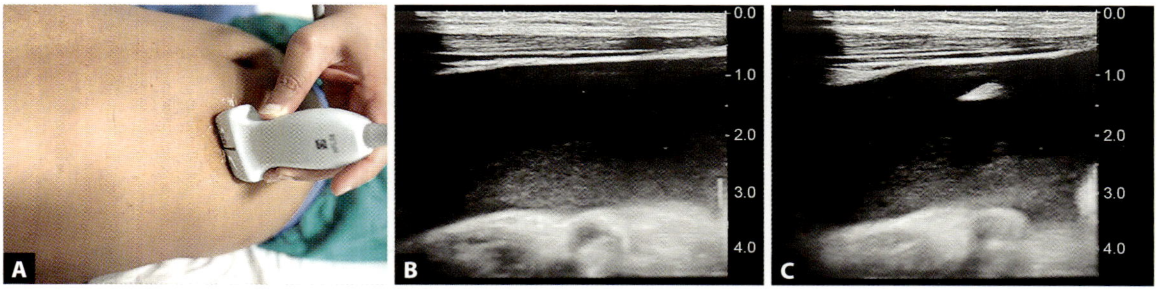

Figs. 11A to C: (A) Probe positioning for ascitic tapping; (B) Ascites view in ultrasound (USG); (C) USG-guided needle insertion for ascitic tapping.

LIMITATIONS OF BEDSIDE ABDOMINAL ULTRASOUND

- It is an operator-dependent procedure which requires proper training and practice.
- Limited field of view compared to CT or MRI especially of the deep-seated visceral structures.
- Nonmodifiable factors of the patient, e.g., obesity, surgical scars, and bowel gas limit the visualization of structures.
- *False negatives:* Small or early-stage pathologies may not be detectable with bedside USG.
- *False positives:* Due to reverberations or obscured images there may be false findings during the scan.
- Fluids cannot be differentiated as urine, blood, ascites, or bile as they all appear anechoic on USG.

CONCLUSION

Bedside abdominal USG is an invaluable tool in the hands of an experienced clinicians, providing rapid and dynamic assessment of abdominal structures. Mastering its use can improve diagnostic accuracy in emergency settings and guide timely interventions. Despite the limitations, it is an essential component of modern clinical practice, particularly when used in conjunction with the art of history taking, clinical examination, other diagnostic modalities, and cognitive acumen.

REFERENCES

1. De Burlet KJ, Ing AJ, Larsen PD, Dennett ER. Systematic review of diagnostic pathways for patients presenting with acute abdominal pain. Int J Qual Health Care. 2018;30:678-83.
2. Myhr K, Sandvic H, Morken T, Hunskaar H. Point of care ultrasonography in Norwegian

out-of-hours primary health care. Scand J Prim Health Care. 2017;35:120-5.

3. Cartwright SL, Knudson MP. Evaluation of acute abdominal pain in adults. Am Fam Physician. 2008;77(7):971-8.
4. AAFP. (2016). Table 12: Clinical Procedures Performed by Physicians at their Practice. [online] Available from https://www.aafp.org/about/dive-into-family-medicine/family-medicine-facts/table12.html [Last accessed August, 2025].
5. Stengel D, Leisterer J, Ferrada P, Ekkernkamp A, Mutze S, Hoenning A. Point-of-care ultrasonography for diagnosing thoracoabdominal injuries in patients with blunt trauma. Cochrane Database Syst Rev. 2018;12(12):CD012669.
6. Mattson B, Dulaimy K. The 4 Quadrants: Acute Pathology in the Abdomen and Current Imaging Guidelines. Semin Ultrasound CT MR. 2017;38(4):414-23.
7. Khan MAB, Abu-Zidan FM. Point-of-care ultrasound for the acute abdomen in the primary health care. Turk J Emerg Med. 2020; 20(1):1-11.
8. Noble VE, Nelson B. Manual of Emergency and Critical Care Ultrasound. Cambridge, UK, MA: Cambridge University Press; 2014.
9. Coppolino F, Gatta G, Di Grezia G, Reginelli A, Iacobellis F, Vallone G, et al. Gastrointestinal perforation: ultrasonographic diagnosis. Crit Ultrasound J. 2013;5 Suppl 1(Suppl 1):S4.
10. Tanner TN, Hall BR, Oran J. neumoperitoneum. Surg Clin North Am. 2018;98(5):915-32.
11. Premkumar M, Karvellas CJ, Kulkarni AV, Bhujade H, Reddy KR. Role of point-of-care ultrasound (POCUS) in clinical hepatology. Hepatology. 2024. Epub ahead of print.
12. Abu-Zidan FM, Cevik AA. Diagnostic point-of-care ultrasound (POCUS) for gastrointestinal pathology: state of the art from basics to advanced. World J Emerg Surg. 2018;13:47.
13. Torres-Macho J, Schutzer CM. Point-of-Care Ultrasound in Clinical Care: Abdomen. Med Clin North Am. 2025;109(1):31-45.
14. Gulati M, Cheng J, Loo JT, Skalski M, Malhi H, Duddalwar V. Pictorial review: Renal ultrasound. Clin Imaging. 2018;51:133-54.
15. Kim SH, Cho JY, Lee HJ, Sung CK, Kim SH. Ultrasound of the urinary bladder, revisited. J Med Ultrasound. 2007;15(2):77-90.
16. Bogusiewicz M. Ultrasound imaging in urogynecology - state of the art 2016. Prz Menopauzalny. 2016;15(3):123-32.
17. Gargani L, Volpicelli G. How I do it: lung ultrasound. Cardiovasc Ultrasound. 2014;12:25.
18. Amini R. Procedural guidance with ultrasound in the emergency patient. Ultrasound Clin. 2014;9(2):217-26.

CHAPTER 7

Musculoskeletal Ultrasound

Pushpraj Singh, Pallav Singh, Pooja Gautam

WHAT YOU WILL LEARN IN THIS CHAPTER?

A. Overview of various applications of musculoskeletal ultrasound in emergency department (ED).

INTRODUCTION

The use of point-of-care ultrasound (POCUS) in diagnosing and managing musculoskeletal complaints continues to expand, driven by its affordability, dynamic imaging capabilities, immediate results, and portability. These features have established ultrasound (USG) as a valuable imaging modality in urgent care settings, emergency departments (EDs), and musculoskeletal care clinics. This chapter explores the application of musculoskeletal USG in assessing articular and periarticular structures, with a focus on identifying mechanical injuries to soft tissues, vasculature and nerves and their brief management in the ED.

WHY USE MUSCULOSKELETAL ULTRASOUND IN EMERGENCY DEPARTMENT?

Musculoskeletal USG offers a versatile and efficient tool for emergency care. It aids in detecting fractures and soft-tissue injuries, facilitates abscess identification and drainage, and enables foreign body localization. Advanced techniques like water-bath USG enhance imaging in specific scenarios. Additionally, it helps to assess vascular and nerve injuries, infections, inflammatory conditions, and soft-tissue masses. USG is also critical for diagnosing compartment syndrome and providing ED-based pain management, making it an indispensable resource in musculoskeletal emergencies.[1]

CLINICAL APPLICATIONS OF MUSCULOSKELETAL ULTRASOUND IN EMERGENCY DEPARTMENT

Fracture Detection

- USG can identify fractures, particularly in cases where X-rays are inconclusive or not immediately available. It is especially useful for detecting fractures in areas like the ribs, clavicle, and small bones **(Fig. 1)**.
- Studies have shown that USG is effective in detecting fractures, especially in pediatric patients where radiation exposure is a concern.[2]

Soft-tissue Injuries

- USG is useful in diagnosing soft-tissue injuries, such as tendon and ligament tears, muscle injuries, and hematomas.[3]

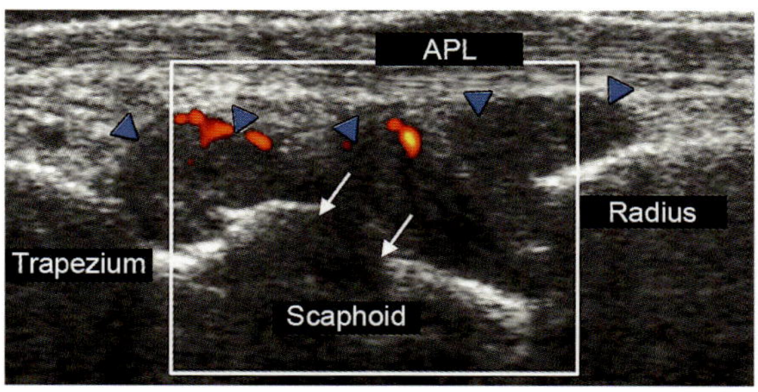

Fig. 1: Scaphoid fracture. Ultrasound (USG) image showing interruption of scaphoid cortex and adjacent hematoma displacing the abductor pollicis longus (APL) tendon.

- Research supports the use of USG in detecting soft-tissue injuries, with high accuracy in diagnosing conditions such as rotator cuff tears **(Fig. 2)** and Achilles tendon **(Figs. 3A and B)** injuries.

Water-bath Ultrasound Technique for Fracture Detection (Figs. 4A to C)[4]

- Water is used as a contrast medium.
- Since water will take up some of the superficial part of the image, the depth of the screen is increased.

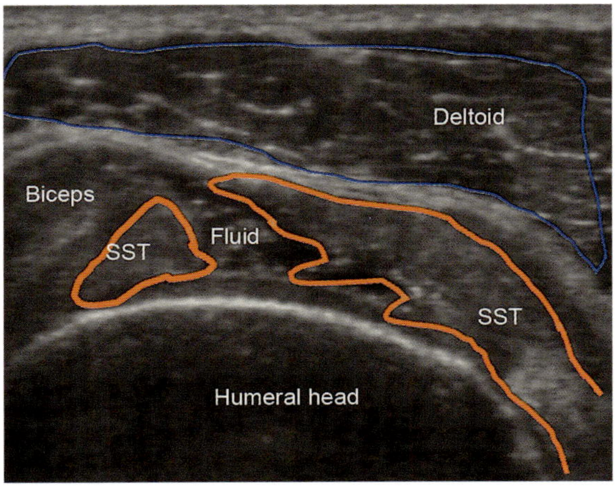

Fig. 2: Tear of midportion of supraspinatus tendon (SST) of rotator cuff. A fluid-filled gap is present withing the tendon.

- The pathological site can be evaluated without touching the patient's skin.
- The superficial structures of interest can be viewed in the focus.
- The water bath used as a medium for sound transmission, enhances the contrast and provides superior diagnostic quality.
- Submerging the patient's extremity in the water bath replaces the need for USG gel or contact between the USG transducer and the patient's skin, thus eliminating discomfort, compression, and distortion of the superficial tissue.

Abscess Identification and Drainage

- USG is crucial in differentiating between cellulitis and abscesses. It also guides the precise drainage of abscesses.[5]
- POCUS is excellent at differentiating a pocket of fluid from tissue edema; however, diagnosis for cellulitis **(Fig. 5)** or abscess should be made keeping in mind the clinical presentation of the patient. The clinical context should support infection, local swelling from an allergic reaction, or more diffuse swelling as seen in congestive heart failure or low serum protein disorders.
- Several studies have demonstrated that USG improves the success rate of abscess drainage and reduces the need for more invasive procedures.

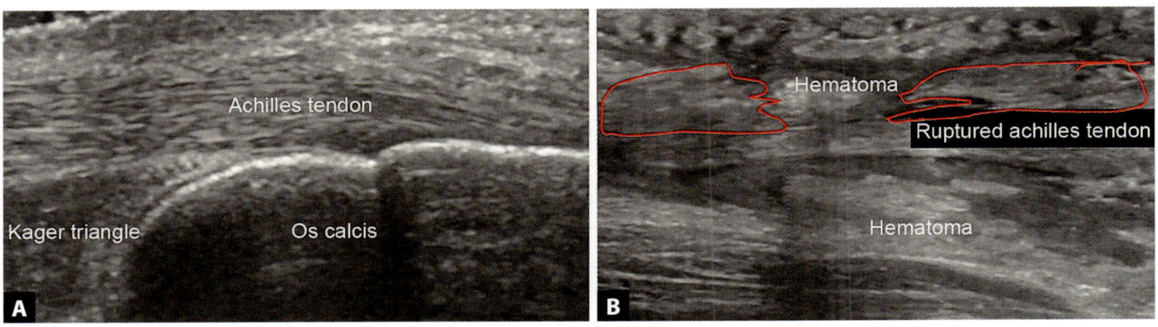

Figs. 3A and B: (A) Normal Achilles tendon on ultrasound (USG); (B) Ruptured tendoachilles with hematoma above and below the tendon.

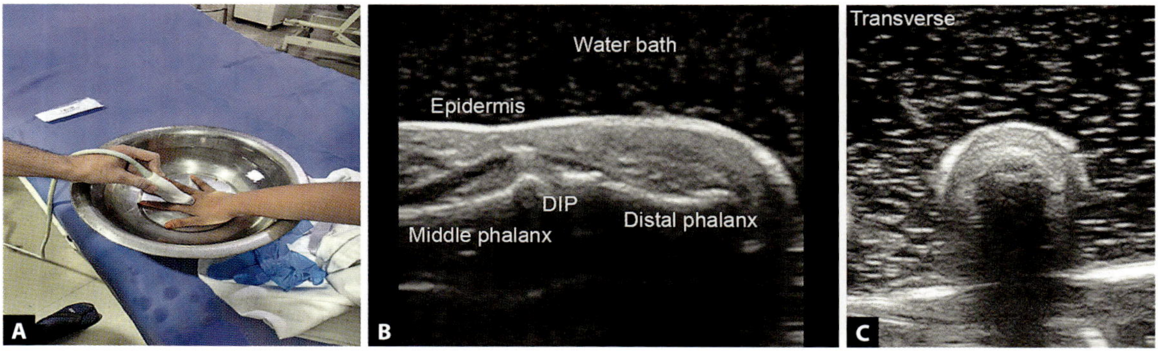

Figs. 4A to C: Water-bath ultrasound technique: Patient's hand placed in warm water, where water is used as a contrast medium if the surface to be scanned is irregular or painful. (DIP: distal interphalangeal joint)

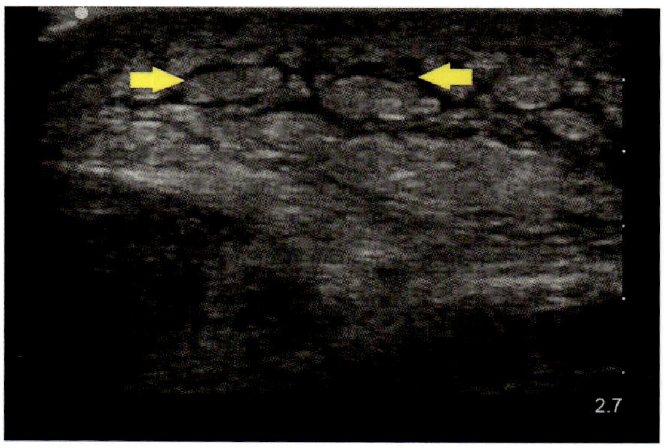

Fig. 5: Cellulitis with cobblestone appearance (yellow arrows).

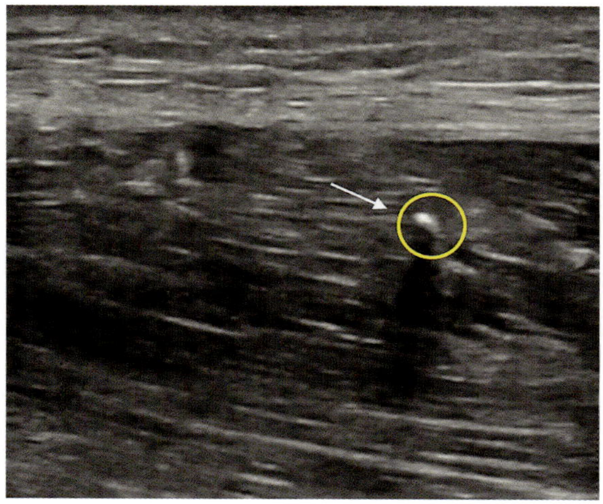

Fig. 6: Broken pacing needle in rectus abdominis muscle (arrow).

Foreign Body Detection[6]

- USG can detect radiolucent foreign bodies (like wood or glass) in soft tissues **(Fig. 6)**.
- Often the bony, articular surfaces may appear hyperechoic, and a small foreign body might be difficult to visualize.
- USG has been shown to be highly effective in localizing and guiding the removal of soft-tissue foreign bodies, improving patient outcomes.

Vascular and Nerve Injuries (Figs. 7A and B)[7]

- USG can detect vascular injuries and help in diagnosing nerve injuries.
- It is increasingly used in the ED for guiding peripheral nerve blocks, providing effective pain relief while minimizing complications.

Infections and Inflammatory Conditions

- USG is valuable in diagnosing infections such as osteomyelitis and septic arthritis, by

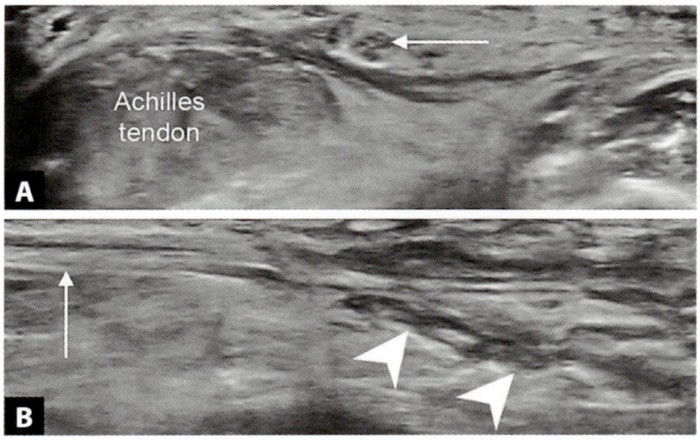

Figs. 7A and B: (A) Arrow indicates the sural nerve in transverse view; (B) Arrow demonstrates the longitudinal course of the sural nerve, while the arrowhead highlights an interruption in its continuity as it extends deeper.

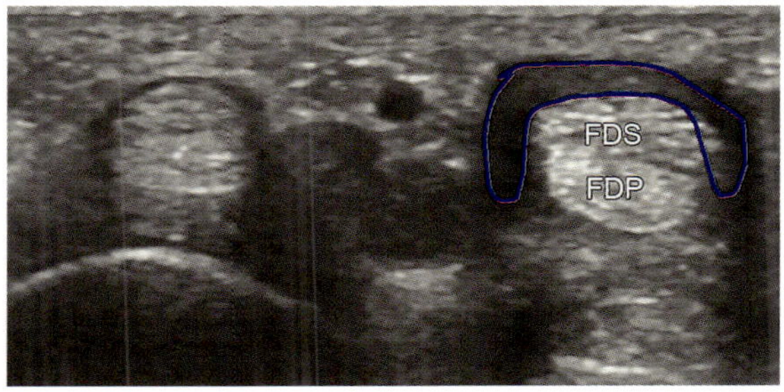

Fig. 8: Transverse section of flexor tenosynovitis. Note the thickened halo around the tendon. (FDP: flexor digitorum profundus; FDS: flexor digitorum superficialis)

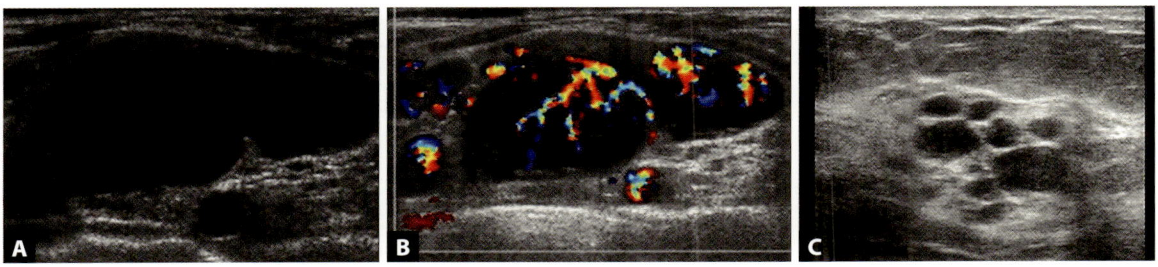

Figs. 9A to C: (A) Supraclavicular lymphoma; (B) Doppler shows vascularity, confirming it as solid mass; (C) Clustered cysts in breast tissue.

identifying signs of inflammation and guiding diagnostic aspirations **(Fig. 8)**.

- Studies have confirmed that it is a reliable tool for early diagnosis of osteomyelitis and septic arthritis, enabling prompt, targeted treatment.[8]

Assessment of Soft-tissue Masses[9]

- USG can be used to assess the nature of soft-tissue masses (cystic vs. solid).
- Real-time-guided biopsy, if needed, can be done using USG **(Figs. 9A to C)**.

Compartment Syndrome

- USG can assist in diagnosing compartment syndrome by measuring compartment thickness and identifying hematomas or muscle edema.
- Though traditionally diagnosed clinically, USG is increasingly recognized for its role in the early diagnosis of compartment syndrome.[10]

Pain Management[11]

- USG is used in the ED to guide nerve blocks for managing acute pain associated with fractures, dislocations, and other injuries.
- USG-guided nerve blocks or fascial plane blocks have brought an evolution in acute pain management with minimal complications.
- The use of USG for guiding regional anesthesia reduces the need for systemic analgesics and improves pain control **(Figs. 10A to D)**.

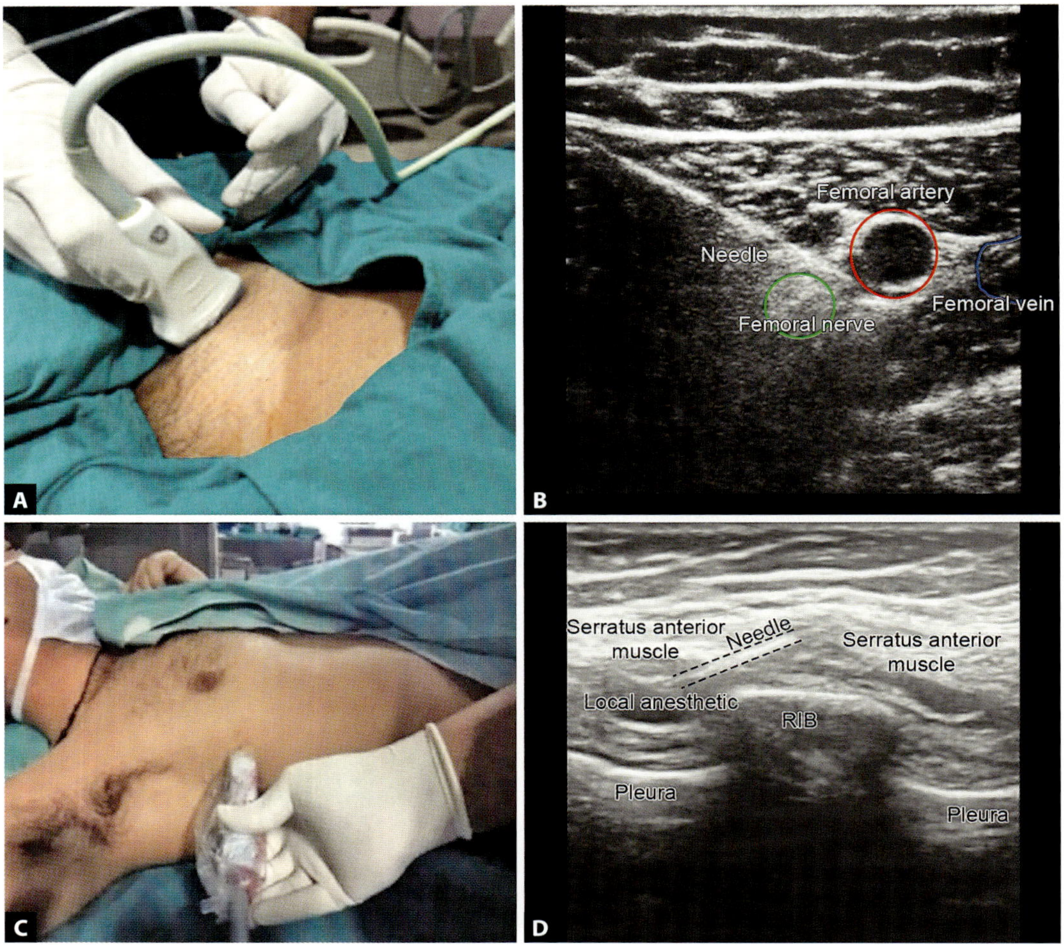

Figs. 10A to D: (A) Needle entry point in long axis to ultrasound (USG) probe; (B) Femoral nerve block; (C) Patient and probe position for serratus anterior plane block; (D) USG image serratus anterior block.

ADVANTAGES OF MUSCULOSKELETAL ULTRASOUND IN THE EMERGENCY DEPARTMENT

- *Bedside accessibility:* Enables faster diagnosis and decision-making at the patient's bedside.
- *Noninvasive and immediate:* Provides rapid and real-time information without the need for more invasive imaging modalities.
- *Both diagnostic and therapeutic:* USG can help in detecting the fractures as well as its reductions in ED. Similarly, an USG comes handy for detection of abscess pocket or foreign body and their drainage/removal.
- *No radiation:* Safe for all patient populations, including children and pregnant women.

LIMITATIONS

- *Operator dependent:* The accuracy of USG depends on the operator's skill and experience.
- *Limited penetration:* There are challenges in imaging deep structures or in patients with a high body mass index.

- *Complex injuries:* More complex injuries may still require CT or MRI for a complete evaluation.

CONCLUSION

Musculoskeletal ultrasound enables rapid, noninvasive and highly effective diagnostic tool for fractures, soft tissue injuries, abscesses and inflammation. It also expedites decision making and enables early guided drainage of abscesses.

USG plays an essential role in optimizing resource allocation and improving workflow efficiency in high-pressure settings.

REFERENCES

1. Zhang M, Xie K. Advances in Musculoskeletal Ultrasound for Assistive Diagnosis in Pain Clinics. Pain Ther. 2025;14(3):791-801.
2. Mobasseri A. Practical strategies to lower radiation exposure in pediatrics distal radius fractures: an orthopedic view. J Orthop Rep. 2024;3(4): 100363.
3. Shah AB, Bhatnagar N. Ultrasound imaging in musculoskeletal injuries—what the orthopaedic surgeon needs to know. J Clin Orthop Trauma. 2019;10(4):659-65. Erratum in: J Clin Orthop Trauma. 2020;11(6):1169-71. Erratum in: J Clin Orthop Trauma. 2021;21:101556.
4. Shrimal P, Bhoi S, Sinha TP, Murmu LR, Nayer J, Ekka M, et al. Sensitivity and specificity of waterbath ultrasound technique in comparison to the conventional methods in diagnosing extremity fractures. Am J Emerg Med. 2022;53:118-21.
5. Squire BT, Fox JC, Anderson C. ABSCESS: applied bedside sonography for convenient evaluation of superficial soft tissue infections. Acad Emerg Med. 2005;12(7):601-6.
6. Blyme PJ, Lind T, Schantz K, Lavard P. Ultrasonographic detection of foreign bodies in soft tissue: a human cadaver study. Arch Orthop Trauma Surg. 1990;110(1):24-5.
7. Nejati A, Teymourian H, Behrooz L, Mohseni G. Pain management via ultrasound-guided nerve block in emergency department: a case series study. Emerg (Tehran). 2017;5(1):e12.
8. Oji NM, Sabatini CS. Osteomyelitis and septic arthritis of the upper extremity in pediatric patients. Curr Rev Musculoskelet Med. 2025;18(3):61-72.
9. Carra BJ, Bui-Mansfield LT, O'Brien SD, Chen DC. Sonography of musculoskeletal soft-tissue masses: techniques, pearls, and pitfalls. AJR Am J Roentgenol. 2014;202(6):1281-90.
10. Mühlbacher J, Pauzenberger R, Asenbaum U, Gauster T, Kapral S, Herkner H, et al. Feasibility of ultrasound measurement in a human model of acute compartment syndrome. World J Emerg Surg. 2019;14:4.
11. Marrone F, Pullano C, De Cassai A, Fusco P. Ultrasound-guided fascial plane blocks in chronic pain: a narrative review. J Anesth Analg Crit Care. 2024;4(1):71.

CHAPTER 8

Vascular Ultrasound

Shyam Sundar, Subhankar Paul, Alka Verma

WHAT YOU WILL LEARN IN THIS CHAPTER?

A. Deep vein thrombosis (DVT) screening in emergency

B. Inferior vena cava (IVC) imaging

C. Abdominal aorta imaging

D. Peripheral arterial Doppler—basics

INTRODUCTION

Why do vascular ultrasound in emergency?

Vascular ultrasound plays a crucial role in managing a patient in emergency and intensive care units (ICUs):

- Vascular access under ultrasound vision in a difficult cannulation situation
- Identifying venous thrombosis
- Inferior vena cava (IVC) assessment for fluid responsiveness or tolerance
- Aorta imaging for aneurysm/dissection
- Peripheral arterial Doppler for acute limb ischemia.

ADVANTAGES OF VASCULAR ULTRASOUND

- Noninvasive and rapid diagnosis
- Quick decision-making
- Cost-effective tool
- Guiding intervention
- No radiation exposure
- Can be performed multiple times on bedside
- Real-time imaging
- Available in every emergency department (ED) and ICUs.

DEEP VEIN THROMBOSIS SCREENING IN EMERGENCY[1]

- Untreated deep vein thrombosis (DVT) in the upper or lower extremities can cause catastrophic events as on dislodgment it may lead to pulmonary thromboembolism.
- Ultrasound evaluates for visible clot—partial or complete occlusion. Color Doppler picks up filing defects and checks whether the vein is fully compressible or not.
- *Indications:*
    - Unilateral lower extremities swelling with or without pain and tenderness
    - Positive Homan sign
    - Suspicion of DVT
    - Evaluate for acute/chronic limb ischemia and severity based on peak systolic velocity (PSV)
- Once DVT is visualized, avoid compressing it, as it may dislodge the clot and lead to pulmonary thromboembolism
- *Principles of DVT scanning in emergency/ICU:*
    - First, we need to differentiate the vein and the artery **(Table 1)**
    - Scan in the appropriate parts and look for normal veins or features of DVT **(Table 2)**

- Echogenic material within the lumen of vessels
- Always compare with adjacent artery
- Do confirm with color Doppler to look for filling defect
- Lack of uniform filling defect—indicates DVT
- False positive if scanned with increased gain (both artery and vein lumen appear echogenic)
- Lymph node mistaken as vein—check with color Doppler, change the axis to longitudinal view **(Fig. 3)**.

LOWER LIMB DEEP VEIN THROMBOSIS SCREENING[1]

- *Scanning procedure:*
  - *Position:* The patient lies supine with head elevated at 30°, knee slightly flexed, and leg externally rotated (frog leg position) **(Fig. 4)**
  - *Transducer*—linear probe with venous preset
  - *Sequence of scanning* ***(Fig. 5)****:*
    - *At saphenofemoral junction:*
      - Start with the probe in the groin crease in a short-axis view with indicator toward right side of the patient
      - Search for the "Mickey Mouse" sign at saphenofemoral junction **(Fig. 6)**
      - Femoral vein and great saphenous vein (GSV) will compress while the femoral artery will not.
      - Avoid compression if visible clot is seen in the vein.
      - Activate color Doppler to look for filling defect
      - Take images before and after compression for documentation
    - *Midthigh level:*
      - Move the probe down to midthigh
      - Apply intermitted and instant compression every 1 cm down the plane to look for thrombus
      - Continue scanning till you reach the knee

TABLE 1: Differentiating feature of vein and artery in ultrasound.

Vein	*Artery*
Anechoic	Anechoic
Thin walled	Thick walled
Compressible	Noncompressible
Respiratory variation may be present	Pulsatile

TABLE 2: Principles of DVT scanning in emergency/ICU.

Sonographic characteristics	*Normal vein*	*DVT*	*Comments*
Compressibility	Fully compressible **(Figs. 1A and B)**	Noncompressible or partially compressible **(Fig. 2)**	• Apply enough pressure to distort artery anatomy • Do not compress if visible clot is noted
Echogenicity	Anechoic	Echogenic lumen	Optimal setting required
Color Doppler	Uniform filling	Filling defect	Angle dependent
Pulse wave Doppler	• Augmentation with calf muscle pressure • Respiratory variation	• No augmentation with calf pressure • Lack of variation	• Difficult and painful to compress • Usually, avoidable

(ICU: intensive care; DVT: deep vein thrombosis)

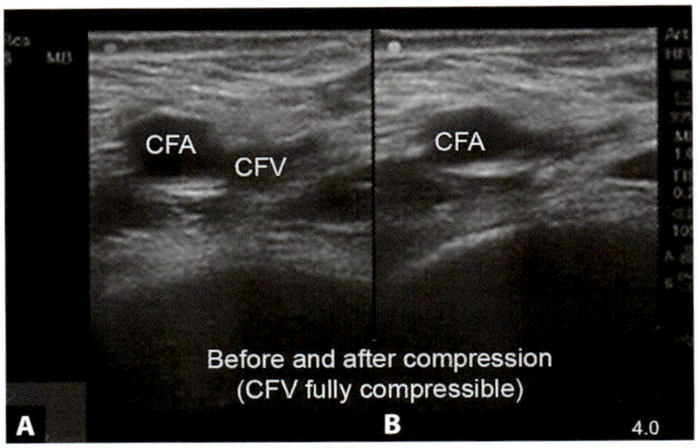

Figs. 1A and B: (A) Before compression; (B) CFV is completely collapsing with compression. (CFA: common femoral artery; CFV: common femoral vein)

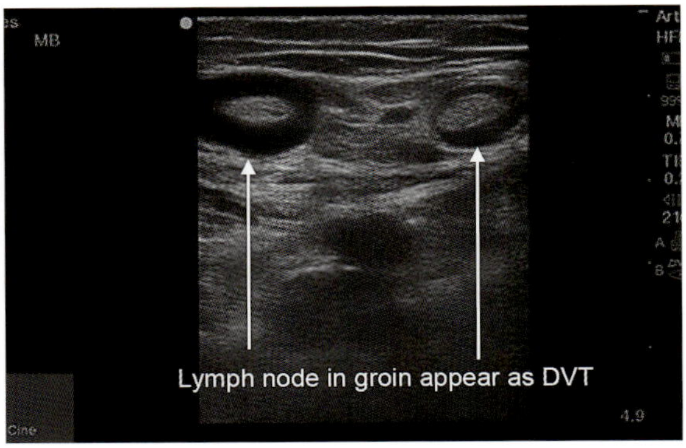

Fig. 3: Lymph node in groin mimicking as deep vein thrombosis (DVT).

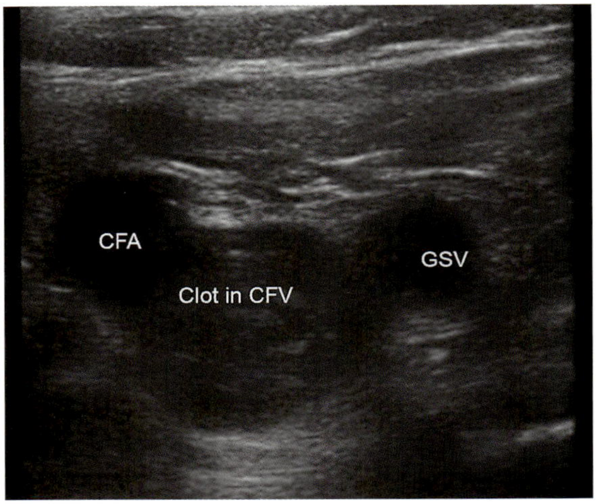

Fig. 2: CFV is not compressible in the presence of a clot within it. (CFA: common femoral artery; CFV: common femoral vein; GSV: great saphenous vein)

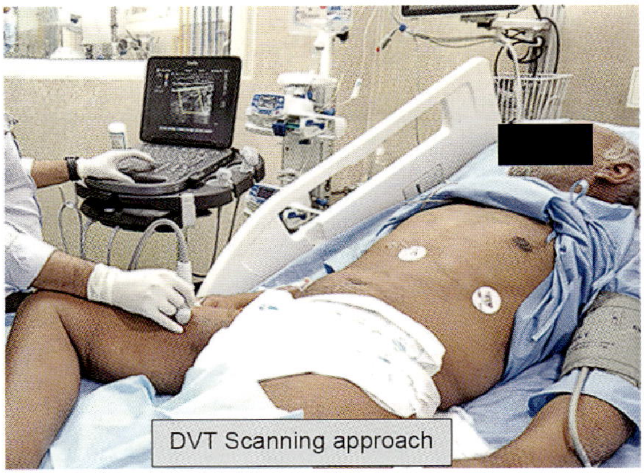

Fig. 4: Positioning of the lower limb for deep vein thrombosis (DVT) screening.

- Rotate the probe 90° from short axis to obtain a longitudinal view to look for even a small thrombus occluding the vein
- *Popliteal fossa:*
  - Scan the popliteal fossa for the popliteal vein (PV) which is lying superficially on the top of the popliteal artery (PA) **(Fig. 7)**
  - Patient will be supine with slight external rotation at the hip joint and knee flexed at 20°
  - Vascular probe faces 9 o'clock for both leg
  - Sweep the probe in craniocaudal direction till you identify PV in the fossa, keep the vein in the center of the screen
  - Apply compressibility test
  - Activate color Doppler
  - Save image before and after compression

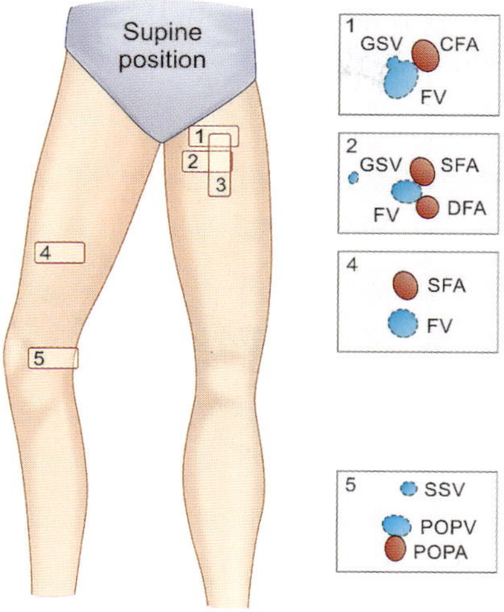

Fig. 5: Steps and probe positioning of screening of deep vein thrombosis (DVT) in lower limb. (CFA: common femoral artery; DFA: deep femoral artery, FV: femoral vein; GSV: great saphenous vein; POPA: popliteal artery; POPV: popliteal vein; SFA: superficial femoral artery; SSV: superficial saphenous vein)

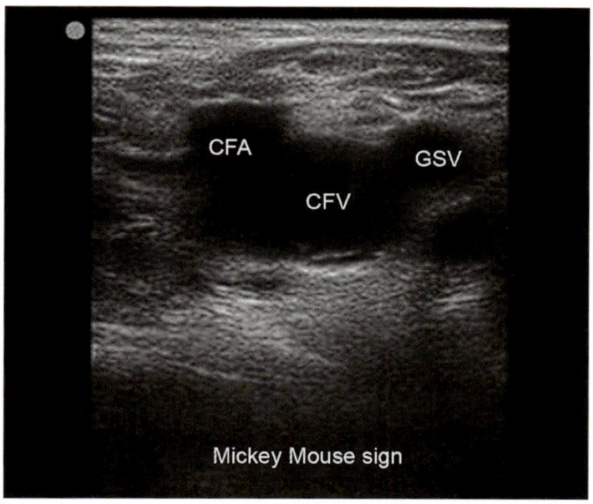

Fig. 6: "Mickey Mouse sign" at groin showing relationship between CFA, CFV, and GSV. (CFA: common femoral artery; CFV: common femoral vein; GSV: great saphenous vein)

- *Two-point compression technique—suitable for emergency physicians:*
  1. Is the FV compressible at saphenofemoral junction?
  2. Is the PV compressible at popliteal fossa?

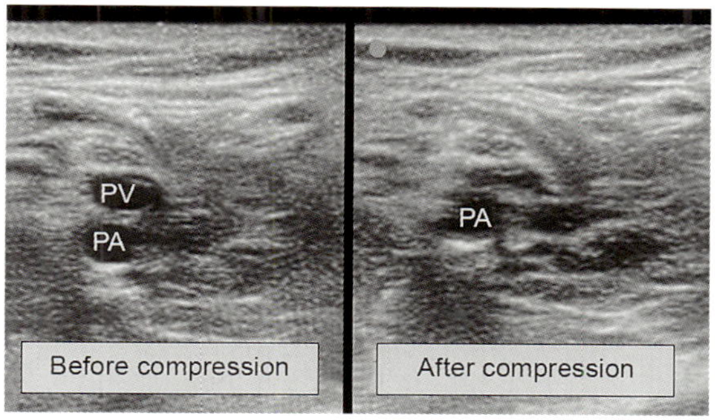

Fig. 7: Popliteal vein (PV) and popliteal artery (PA) in the popliteal fossa.

- *Noncompressible vein:* First differential is DVT.
- *Pitfalls of DVT screening in emergency:*
  - Compressing pressure is not enough leading to interpretation of noncompressibility
  - Probe not centrally placed on vein
  - Artery mistaken as vein
  - Lymph node mistaken as vein
- *Tips:*
  - Keep the area of interest (vein) in middle of the ultrasound screen
  - First, confirm if the structure is an artery or vein.
  - Image the structure in two perpendicular planes (longitudinal and transverse). Lymph nodes remain circular in both planes.

INFERIOR VENA CAVA[2]

- *Indications of scanning:*
  - Undifferentiated shock
  - Fluid responsiveness/fluid tolerance
  - Differentiate various causes of breathlessness
- *Technique (**Fig. 8**):*
  - Patient lies supine with the head end slightly elevated and knee flexed
  - Apply adequate jelly
  - Use a curvilinear/echo probe

- Place the probe in subcostal view, marker pointing toward the head. Slight manipulation of the probe gives a good view of IVC opening into right atrium (RA)→ press M-mode to measure its diameter and respiratory variation **(Figs. 9A and B)**.

- *Reasons for incorrect IVC assessment:*
  - Sometimes aorta can be confused for IVC
  - Ensure IVC is viewed in the full longitudinal axis, off center gives a false lower value
  - Not measuring IVC 0.5 cm proximal to hepatic vein

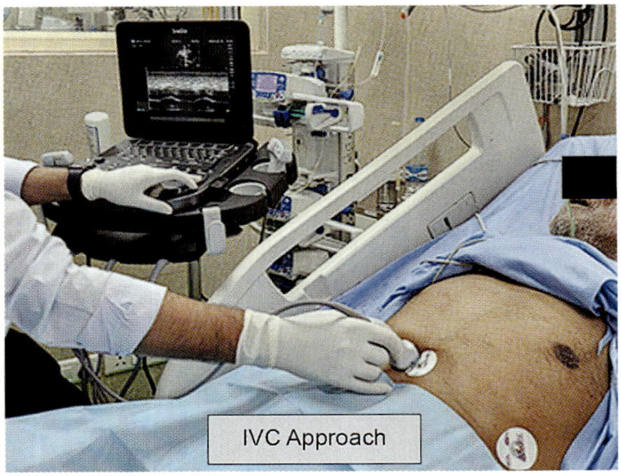

Fig. 8: Technique and probe positioning for inferior vena cava (IVC) measurement.

- With the help of IVC, we can estimate RA pressure in a spontaneously breathing patient. Its diameter decreases with inspiration. The diameter and degree of collapsibility of IVC gives an idea of RA pressure **(Table 3)**.

ABDOMINAL AORTA IMAGING[3]

- Abdominal aorta (AA) is a retroperitoneal organ
- Normal size <3 cm
- *Indications of scanning:*
  - Abdominal aortic aneurysm (AAA)
  - Aortic dissection

    Note: Type 2 can be picked up with 2D echocardiography.
- *Technique:*
  - *Patient positioning:* Supine and flat with slight flexion at the knee joint, like position during IVC imaging
  - *Transducer*—low frequency, curvilinear probe, set mode to abdomen scan
  - Displace the bowel gas by applying firm pressure over abdominal wall
  - Place the probe just below the xiphoid in transverse plane; mild compression will lead to visualization of the vertebral body with IVC and aorta anterior to it. Keep scanning caudally a cm or two till

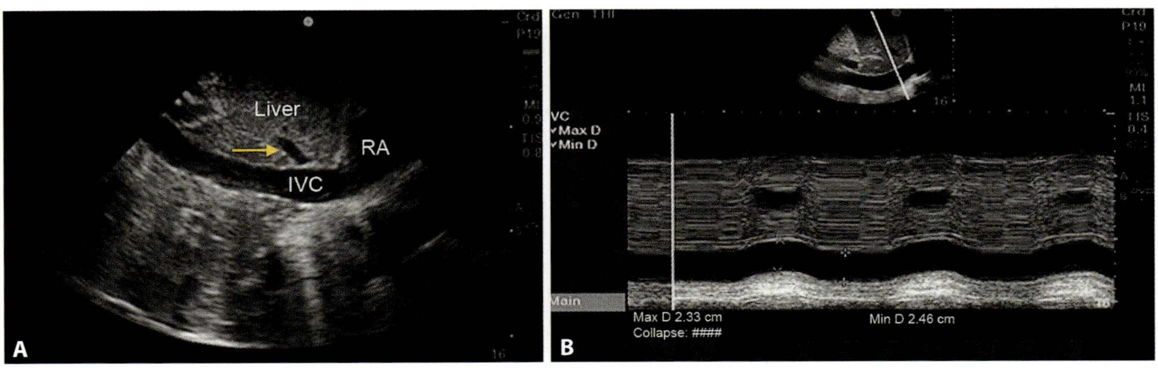

Figs. 9A and B: (A) Inferior vena cava (IVC) in USG 2D-mode, showing the course of IVC through liver and opening into right atrium (RA), hepatic vein (yellow arrow) can also be seen draining into IVC; (B) IVC measurement in M-mode.

TABLE 3: Estimated RA pressure according to IVC size and collapsibility.

IVC size	*IVC collapse during inspiration*	*Estimated RA pressure*	*Comment*
<21 mm	>50%	<5 mm Hg	Normal
<21 mm	<50%	5–10 mm Hg	Intermediate
>21 mm	>50%	5–10 mm Hg	Intermediate
>21 mm	<50%	>10 mm Hg	High

(IVC: inferior vena cava; RA: right atrium)

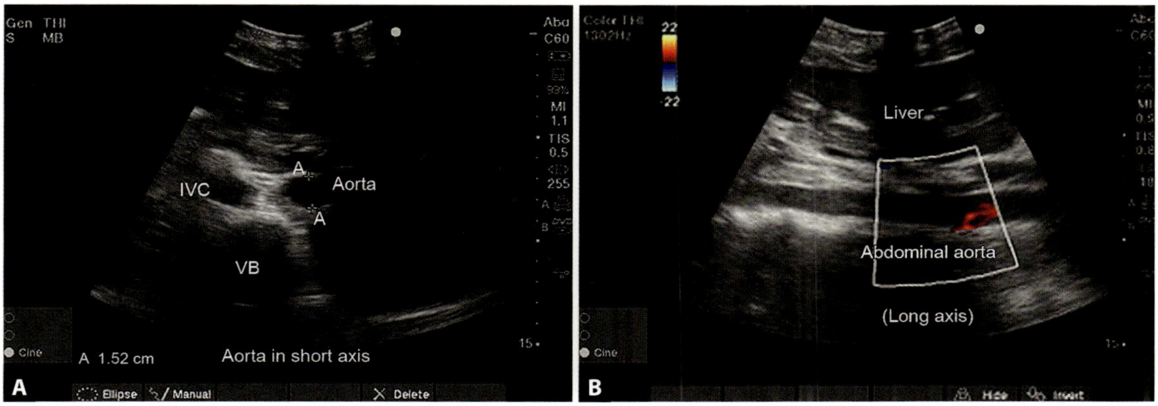

Figs. 10A and B: Abdominal aorta in short axis (left) and long axis (right). (IVC: inferior vena cava; VB: vertebral body)

bifurcation of aorta into iliac arteries is visible

- Attempt to visualize the AA in both sections (short and long axis) **(Figs. 10A and B)**
- Try to identify celiac trunk and superior mesenteric artery
- Save the images and measure size
- Measure the size of aorta from outer-to-outer wall edge and look for focal or diffuse dilatation and flat or false lumen
- If AAA is found, measure the diameter in both axes to look for impending rupture
- If AA diameter is >5.5 cm in size, there is a higher chance of rupture
- Try to identify any dissection flap in the appropriate scenario **(Figs. 11A and B)**.

PERIPHERAL ARTERIAL DOPPLER[4]

- *Indications:*
  - Peripheral arterial disease (critical limb ischemia and intermittent claudication)
  - Traumatic vascular injury
  - Raynaud's phenomenon
- *Scanning tips:*
  - Adequate exposure of the affected limb
  - Select linear probe (5–10 MHz, set vascular mode on ultrasound)
  - Locate the artery with the help of landmark, use B-mode
  - Place the transducer at a 45-to-60° angle to the artery
  - Adjust gain and frequency
  - Evaluate flow pattern

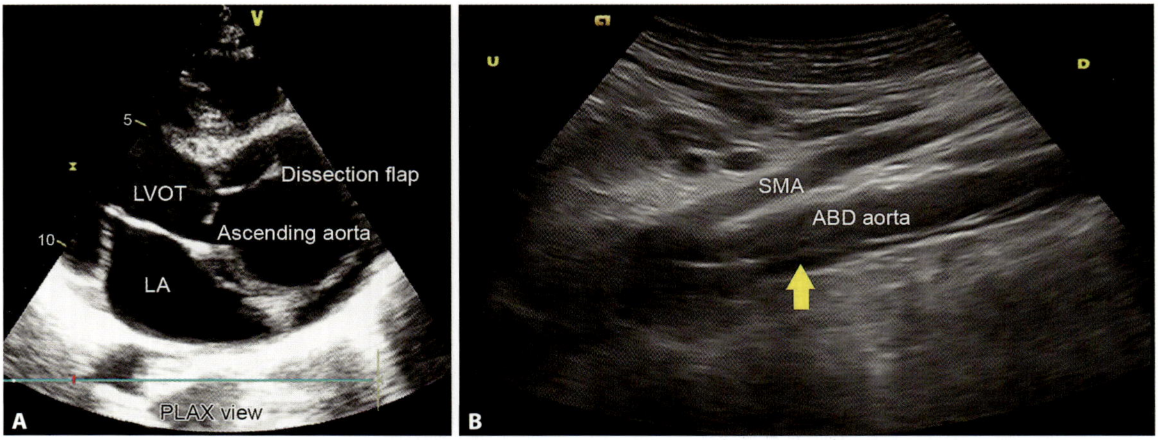

Figs. 11A and B: (A) Aortic dissection flap is seen in ascending aorta in cardiac PLAX view (left); (B) Dissection flap in abdominal aorta (yellow arrow) in abdominal longitudinal view (right). (LA: left atrium; LVOT: left ventricular outflow tract; PLAX: parasternal long axis; SMA: superior mesenteric artery)

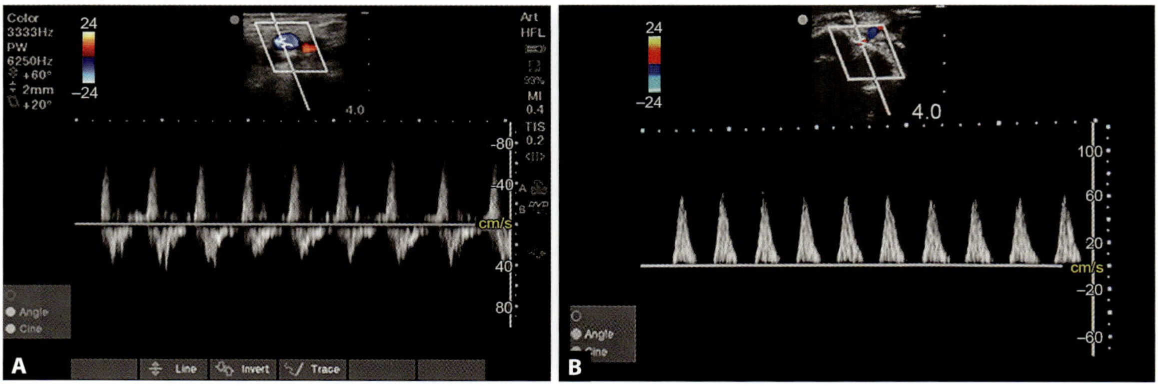

Figs. 12A and B: (A) Triphasic flow (left); (B) Monophasic flow.

- Scan the artery in multiple segments (proximal, mid, and distal)
- Check types of flow and measure velocity
- Obtained two values—PSV and end-diastolic velocity (EDV) [machine calculates resistive index (RI) and pulsatility index (PI)]
- Save the images for documentation
- May repeat if necessary

- *Types of flow in arterial scan:*
  - *Triphasic flow—normal flow pattern in a peripheral artery* ***(Fig. 12A)****:*
    - Forward flow in systole
    - Brief reversal in early diastole
    - Forward flow in late diastole
  - *Biphasic flow—abnormal flow seen in mild stenosis:*
    - Forward flow in systole
    - Brief reversal in early diastole
  - *Monophonic flow—seen in severe stenosis or occlusion* ***(Fig. 12B)****:*
    - Only forward flow throughout the cardiac cycle
  - *Trades parvus flow—proximal stenosis:*
    - Delayed systolic upstroke
    - Reduced peak velocity

TABLE 4: Normal values in peripheral artery.

Characteristics	*PSV (peak systolic velocity)*	*EDV (end-diastolic velocity)*	*RI (resistive index)*	*PI (pulsatility index)*	*Flow*
Normal	60–120 cm/s	10–30 cm/s	0.7–1	1–2	Triphasic
Stenosis	>180 cm/s	>40 cm/s	<0.5	<0.5	Biphasic
Occlusion	No flow detected				Monophasic
Reversal of flow	EDV in negative values				

- *Damped flow—distal occlusion:*
  - Prolonged systolic sunstroke
  - Reduced peak velocity
  - Waveforms can sometimes occur below the baseline
- **Table 4** summarizes different flow characteristics of arterial Doppler in normal and pathological conditions.

CONCLUSION

- Vascular ultrasound plays an important role in emergency department—particularly in patients with shock, hypertensive crisis, or severe shortness of breath.
- Vascular access using ultrasound has become now standard of care in emergency and critical care settings.
- Trainees need to practice to learn the art of vascular ultrasound as it has a learning curve.

REFERENCES

1. Fox JC, Bertoglio KC. Emergency physician performed ultrasound for DVT evaluation. Thrombosis. 2011;2011(1):938709.
2. Spiliotaki E, Saranteas T, Moschovaki N, Panagouli K, Pistioli E, Kitsinelis V, et al. Inferior vena cava ultrasonography in the assessment of intravascular volume status and fluid responsiveness in the emergency department and intensive care unit: a critical analysis review. J Clin Ultrasound. 2022;50(5):733-44.
3. Rubano E, Mehta N, Caputo W, Paladino L, Sinert R. Systematic review: emergency department bedside ultrasonography for diagnosing suspected abdominal aortic aneurysm. Academic Emerg Med. 2013;20(2):128-38.
4. Kim ES, Sharma AM, Scissons R, Dawson D, Eberhardt RT, Gerhard-Herman M, et al. Interpretation of peripheral arterial and venous Doppler waveforms: a consensus statement from the Society for Vascular Medicine and Society for Vascular Ultrasound. Vasc Med. 2020;25(5):484-506.

CHAPTER 9

Ultrasound-guided Emergency Procedures

Prem Raj Singh, Alka Verma, Divya Srivastava, Shefali Gautam

WHAT YOU WILL LEARN IN THIS CHAPTER?

A. Step-by-step guidance on ultrasound (USG)-guided procedures in emergency department

B. USG-guided cricothyroidotomy, airway management, vascular access, and pleural and pericardial effusion tapping

INTRODUCTION

Ultrasound (USG), once used exclusively as a diagnostic tool, has now become an indispensable part of almost every clinical specialty. Many medical or interventional procedures are now conducted safely by real-time visualizations using ultrasonography. In emergency and critical care settings, bedside USG-guided procedures have been rapidly growing, along with the rise of point-of-care ultrasound (POCUS). Since the initial use of USG to guide pericardiocentesis in the 1990s, many procedures have been developed and popularized in emergency and urgent care settings using real-time USG images. This chapter systematically introduces such procedures with tips and tricks, along with some technical details and troubleshooting for novice practitioners. Indications, contraindications, and preparations needed for USG-guided procedures are mentioned in **Tables 1 and 2**.

CRICOTHYROIDOTOMY

In situations where intubation fails, an emergency cricothyrotomy (making an incision in the throat to create an airway) might be necessary. USG can help to identify the important structures and guide this procedure as well.

- Surgical cricothyroidotomy is a procedure to establish an airway by creating a direct

TABLE 1: Indications and contraindications for ultrasound-guided procedures.

Procedure	*Indications*	*Contraindications*
Central venous access	Emergency vascular access, vasopressors/inotropes administration	Active local infection, thrombosis at access site
Cricothyroidotomy	Airway obstruction, failed intubation	Anatomical abnormalities, age under 12 years
Arterial cannulation	Continuous arterial pressure monitoring, ABG sampling	Severe peripheral vascular disease, coagulopathy
Thoracentesis	Pleural effusion, dyspnea	Unstable patient, coagulation disorders
Pericardiocentesis	Cardiac tamponade, large pericardial effusion	Uncorrected bleeding disorders, aortic dissection

TABLE 2: Equipment checklist for ultrasound-guided procedures.

Item	*Purpose/usage*	*Procedure examples*
Ultrasound machine	Provides real-time imaging guidance	All ultrasound-guided procedures
High-frequency linear transducer	High-resolution imaging of superficial structures	Central venous access, cricothyroidotomy
Phased array transducer	Imaging deeper structures like the heart	Pericardiocentesis
Sterile gel	Ensures good contact between transducer and skin	All procedures
Sterile sheath	Covers the transducer to maintain a sterile field	All procedures
Needle (appropriate gauge)	Insertion into vessels or cavities	Central venous access, thoracentesis
Guidewire	Facilitates catheter placement	Central venous access, cricothyroidotomy
Catheter	Establishes a secure line for fluid administration	Central venous access, arterial cannulation
Scalpel	Used for initial incision	Cricothyroidotomy
Syringe	For aspiration of fluids	Thoracentesis, pericardiocentesis

incision into the cricothyroid membrane and cannulating the trachea. It is indicated when:

- There is a failure to secure an airway in a timely manner.
- There is inadequate or impossible ventilation after detachment from a ventilator.
- As an emergency failsafe measure in "cannot intubate, cannot ventilate" situation during or after administration of general anesthesia.[1]

- Cricothyroidotomy is best avoided in children younger than 12 years old due to the anatomical positioning of the cricothyroid membrane. Transtracheal jet ventilation or needle cricothyrotomy are preferred instead.
- Utilizing real-time ultrasonography leads to better puncture accuracy than marking the skin after static capture of cricothyroid membrane images.[2]

Five key steps to perform ultrasound-guided cricothyroidotomy:

1. *Patient positioning and preparation:* Position the patient supine with the neck extended (if possible) to better expose the cricothyroid membrane. Use a rolled towel under the shoulders to extend the neck. Ensure proper hand hygiene, apply antiseptic to the neck, and drape the area to maintain a sterile field.
2. *Ultrasound examination:* Use a high-frequency linear transducer to identify the relevant neck structures, including the thyroid cartilage, cricoid cartilage, and the cricothyroid membrane, which lies between them. Confirm the position of the cricothyroid membrane in both transverse and longitudinal views, marking the membrane's location on the skin.

3. *Marking the insertion site:* Once the cricothyroid membrane is identified and confirmed, mark the site directly over the membrane where the incision will be made. This marking will guide the incision and needle placement during the procedure **(Figs. 1A and B)**.
4. *Incision and needle insertion:* Make a vertical or horizontal incision over the cricothyroid membrane with a scalpel. Under continuous ultrasound guidance, insert the needle into the cricothyroid membrane at the marked site. Advance the needle until it enters the trachea, confirmed by air aspiration or visualization on ultrasound.
5. *Dilator and tube insertion:* After needle placement, introduce a guidewire through the needle into the trachea. Remove the needle while leaving the guidewire in place. Using the Seldinger technique, pass a dilator over the guidewire to enlarge the opening, then advance the cricothyroidotomy tube (or an appropriately sized endotracheal tube) into the trachea. Confirm tube placement with ultrasound, auscultation, or end-tidal CO_2 monitoring, then secure the tube in place and ventilate the patient.

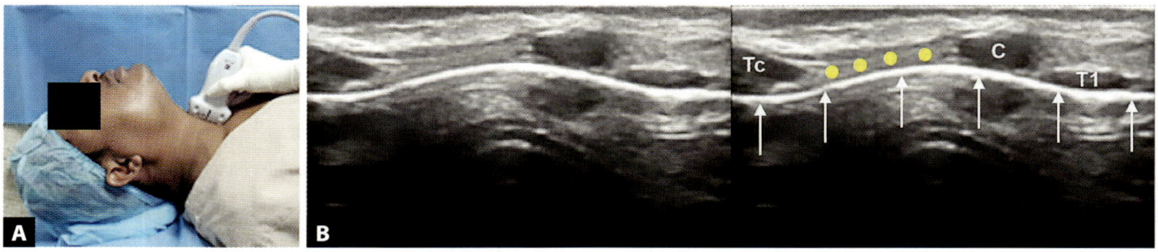

Figs. 1A and B: (A) Probe placement for cricothyroid membrane; (B) Sonographic view showing cricothyroid membrane between thyroid and cricoid cartilage. (Arrows: air-mucosal interface; C: cricoid cartilage; Tc: thyroid cartilage; T1: first tracheal ring; Yellow dots: cricothyroid membrane)

VASCULAR ACCESS: CENTRAL AND PERIPHERAL

- Establishing vascular access is of utmost importance in emergency situations. Emergencies such as respiratory collapse, cardiovascular shock, or sudden/uncontrollable bleeding need immediate intravenous access most often in patients with collapsed untraceable veins.
- There are two approaches to achieve vascular access: (1) Peripheral and (2) central. Literature shows that bedside USG imaging could significantly improve the success rate of peripheral intravenous (PIV) cannulation in the emergency department (ED) population.[3]

Ultrasound-guided Central Venous Access (Figs. 2 to 5)

- Central venous catheter (CVC) access can be achieved through one of the three main veins, (1) the internal jugular (IJ), (2) subclavian (SC), and (3) femoral veins.
- USG is especially useful for IJ access because the landmarks are not always clear (as in thick neck individuals), anatomy can vary, and there are no bones obstructing the view. It is also the most studied and considered safer than doing a blind SC approach.
- For the SC, USG can assist with a supraclavicular approach or help with accessing the axillary vein further down.

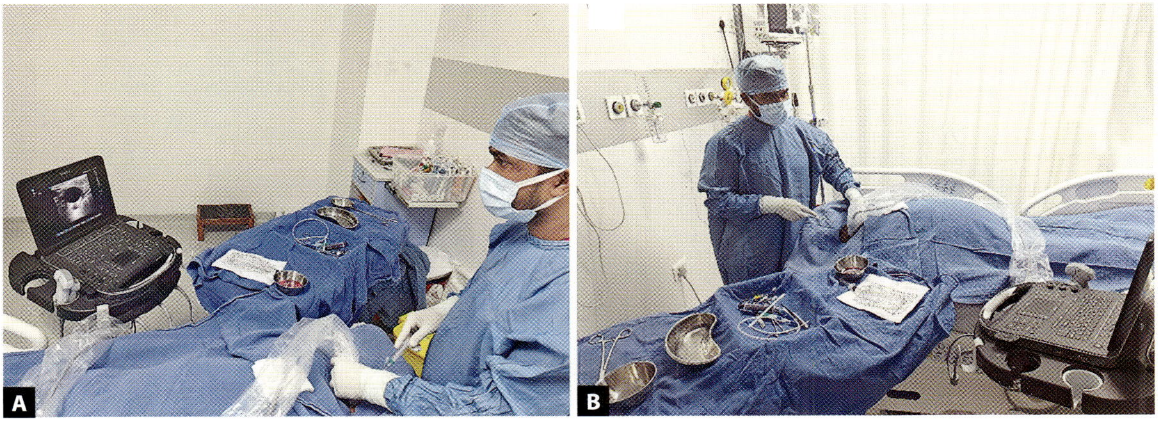

Figs. 2A and B: Positioning and ergonomics for USG-guided CVC insertion in right IJV. *Note:* USG machine should be placed in the same side and in front of the eyes and screen preferably in the same plane of the eyes of the operator. (CVC: central venous catheter; IJV: internal jugular vein; USG: ultrasound)

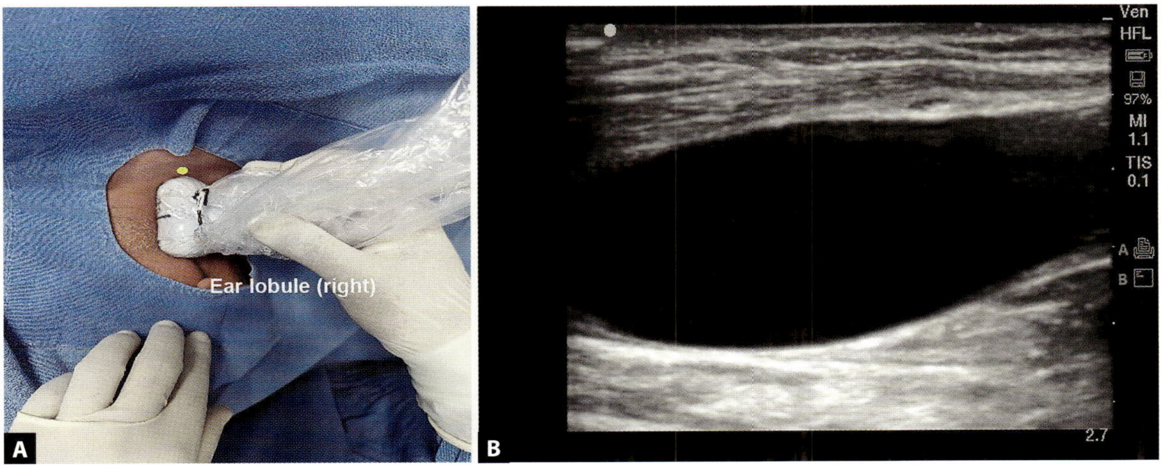

Figs. 3A and B: Probe positioning and USG images of in-plane approach of CVC insertion. Note the probe pointer positioning (yellow dot). (CVC: central venous catheter; USG: ultrasound)

- Although the femoral vein is not ideal for routine use due to higher infection and complication risks, it might be the most accessible during emergencies, and ultrasonic visualization of femoral artery and vein help in such situations.
- Before starting the procedure, if time allows, the target vessel should be scanned both cranially and caudally to check for any abnormalities like unusual anatomy, valves, scars, or clots. The vein should be clear and compressible.
- After sterile draping, local anesthetic, mostly 2% lignocaine is infiltrated around the expected site of puncture.
- For best results, it is recommended to use a dynamic, in-plane long-axis (LAX) approach with one person controlling the USG. This way, the entire needle can be seen during insertion, reducing the risk of placing it

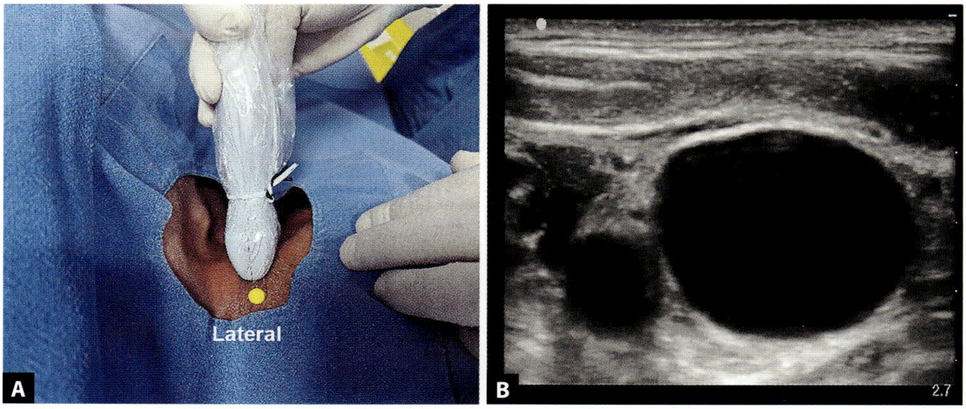

Figs. 4A and B: Probe positioning and USG images of out-of-plane approach of CVC insertion. Note the probe pointer positioning (yellow dot). (CVC: central venous catheter; USG: ultrasound)

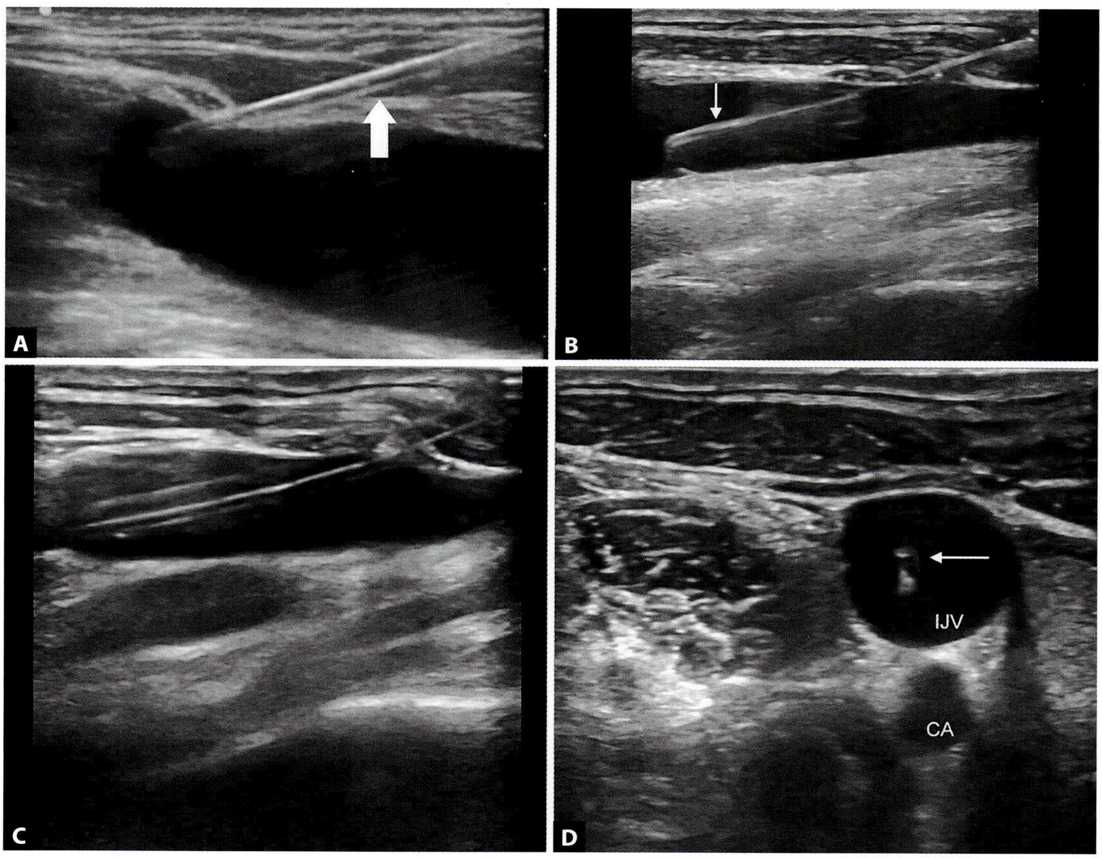

Figs. 5A to D: (A) Insertion of needle (up arrow) in in-plane approach; (B) Insertion of guidewire (down arrow) under vision; (C) Position of guidewire after placement in longitudinal view; (D) Short axis view of guidewire in the IJV lumen. (CA: carotid artery; IJV: internal jugular vein)

incorrectly. However, it can also be helpful to start out in the short-axis (SAX) (out-of-plane) to make sure you are targeting the vein and not the artery, and that you are approaching the center of the vessel. Switching between SAX and LAX views can help confirm that you are working with the vein, not the artery.

- Needling of the target vein is done in real time under ultrasonic visualization. Once the position of the needle is confirmed both by image on screen and by "flash" of blood, then the USG probe is set aside and the guidewire introduced through the needle. The wire is revisualized and its position inside the vein confirmed in both longitudinal and transverse plane. This is followed by dilation and railroading of catheter over the guidewire.
- USG can also help to spot issues like valves that might block the guidewire, help to reposition it, if needed. USG can also be used to confirm the tip of IJ and SC catheter by visualizing bubbles in the right heart during an intravenous flush through the catheter. Lungs are also scanned to rule out pneumothorax, a complication that might occur in SC, axillary, or low IJ cannulations.
- Training with USG for vascular access can improve skills and reduce mistakes.

Five key steps to perform ultrasound-guided internal jugular cannulation:

1. *Patient positioning and preparation:* Position the patient supine with a slight Trendelenburg tilt (head down) to distend the central veins and reduce the risk of air embolism. Turn the patient's head slightly away from the insertion site to improve access. Ensure proper hand hygiene, prepare the skin with antiseptic, and drape the area to maintain a sterile field.
2. *Ultrasound examination:* Use a high-frequency linear transducer to identify the target vein. Scan the area in both transverse (short-axis) and longitudinal (long-axis) views to assess vein size, depth, and patency, and to ensure no nearby arteries or other structures will be accidentally punctured.
3. *Marking the insertion site:* Once the target vein is identified, compress the vein with the transducer to confirm its compressibility (to distinguish it from arteries) and mark the optimal insertion point on the skin.
4. *Needle insertion and cannulation:* Administer local anesthesia at the marked site. Under continuous ultrasound guidance, insert the needle into the skin at a shallow angle, visualizing the needle tip as it enters the vein. Once the needle is in the vein, confirm proper placement by visualizing a flash of blood and then advance a guidewire through the needle. After securing the guidewire, remove the needle and proceed with catheter placement over the guidewire, using the Seldinger technique.
5. *Confirmation and securing the catheter:* After placing the catheter, confirm its position by aspirating blood from each lumen and flushing with saline. Use ultrasound to visualize the guidewire or catheter within the vein to ensure it has not migrated. Secure the catheter with sutures or a sterile adhesive device and apply a sterile dressing. A chest X-ray may be performed to confirm the final position and to rule out complications such as pneumothorax.

Ultrasound-guided Peripheral Venous Access

- Getting PIV access in the emergency department is essential for patient care, for administration of fluids and medications.
- Traditionally, PIV access is achieved by feeling for veins and visually locating them, using tools such as needles and angiocatheters. While this method works in most cases, it can be challenging for certain patients, such

as those with a history of IV drug abuse, chemotherapy, or those on dialysis. When standard PIV access is difficult, other options include placing a cannula in the external jugular vein, using intraosseous lines, PICC lines, or, if necessary, CVCs are used. However, these alternatives can take more time and have risks more than benefit.

- USG can make the process of cannulation easier, much like it does with central venous catheterization. It can help to locate veins that are deeper and not easily found by touch or sight. Using similar techniques as for USG-guided central line placement, medical providers can access peripheral veins more reliably, ensuring better stability of the IV line.
- *Indications:*
  - The reasons for using USG to guide PIV access are the same as for traditional PIV cannulation—it allows access to the bloodstream for blood draws, medication administration, fluids in emergencies, and even short-term nutrition.
  - USG has proven to increase success rates in patients who have difficult venous access, such as those with obesity, history of IV drug abuse, patients undergoing chemotherapy, those with advanced kidney disease and patients after prolonged hospitalization.

ARTERIAL CANNULATION

- Arterial cannulation can be safely and effectively performed under USG guidance. Among vascular access procedures, arterial cannulation is the most technically demanding and associated with adverse effects.
- The radial, ulnar, and brachial arteries in the upper extremities, as well as the dorsalis pedis, posterior tibial, and femoral arteries in the lower extremities, are commonly used for arterial catheterization. To visualize these arteries, a high-frequency linear transducer or hockey stick transducer (especially useful in pediatric patients) is typically used.
- Duplex ultrasonography and color Doppler can help to detect arterial pulses.
- Always perform a modified Allen's test before radial artery cannulation
- There are two main USG-guided techniques: (1) The SAX out-of-plane approach and (2) the LAX in-plane approach. Both approaches have shown similar success rates for radial artery cannulation in adults and children, with some studies also suggesting an oblique approach.[4]

Five key steps to perform ultrasound-guided arterial cannulation ***(Figs. 6 and 7)***

1. *Patient positioning and preparation:* Position the patient comfortably with the target artery exposed. For radial artery cannulation, the patient's arm should be extended with the wrist slightly dorsiflexed (about 30°). Ensure proper hand hygiene and prepare the skin with an antiseptic solution. Drape the area to maintain a sterile field.
2. *Ultrasound examination:* Use a high-frequency linear transducer to identify the target artery (commonly the radial, femoral, or brachial artery). Scan the artery in both transverse (short-axis) and longitudinal (long-axis) views to assess its size, depth, and course. Confirm the absence of any surrounding structures (e.g., veins or nerves) that could complicate the procedure. Check for compressibility to differentiate the artery from veins.
3. *Marking the insertion site:* Once the artery is clearly visualized, mark the optimal insertion point on the skin. For radial artery cannulation, this is typically 1–2 cm proximal to the wrist crease.

4. *Needle insertion:* Under continuous ultrasound guidance, insert the needle at a shallow angle to the skin, either in-plane (long-axis) or out-of-plane (short-axis) depending on the operator's preference and skill level. Visualize the needle tip entering the arterial lumen on the ultrasound screen. You will get a pulsatile flash back of blood when the needle is correctly positioned within the artery.
5. *Catheter advancement and securing:* Once arterial blood return is seen, advance the guidewire (if using the Seldinger technique) or the catheter into the artery while holding the needle steady. After successful cannulation, secure the catheter in place with sterile adhesive or sutures, and apply a sterile dressing. Confirm arterial waveform on a pressure transducer or by blood gas analysis to ensure proper placement.

THORACENTESIS

- A chest radiograph is typically the first imaging choice to detect pleural effusion, but it has its limitations. For instance, a lateral upright chest X-ray requires at least 50 mL of fluid to detect a pleural effusion, while a standard posterior-anterior chest X-ray might only show signs like blunting of the costophrenic recesses and diaphragm obliteration when there is 200–500 mL of fluid. Additionally, a supine anterior-posterior chest X-ray can sometimes miss even significant amounts of fluid.
- In contrast, transthoracic ultrasound (TUS) has several advantages, including no radiation exposure, low cost, portability, and the ability to be used at the bedside.
- TUS has gained popularity among pulmonologists and intensivists for evaluating pleuropulmonary conditions and is now considered the "gold standard" for detecting pleural effusion. It can identify fluid volumes as small as 10 mL, making it far more sensitive than standard chest X-rays.[5]
- In cases where a chest X-ray shows a white hemithorax, TUS can help to differentiate between effusion and lung consolidations, confirming or ruling out massive effusion.
- While TUS can suggest the nature of the pleural fluid, a definitive diagnosis usually requires thoracentesis for further analysis.
- For USG-guided pleural pigtail insertion, place patient in supine position, using curvilinear probe, either in transverse or longitudinal view, look for anechoic (dark) fluid collection between lung and chest wall. In case of massive effusions lung can be seen floating as bright echogenic substance with the fluid. Quantify the volume of fluid in transverse view by the Balik formula.
- Volume of fluid (mL) = maximum distance between pleural and visceral pleura [known as pleural line to lung distance (PLLD)] × 20 **(Fig. 8)**.
- Identify maximum point of separation between lung and chest wall, and insert a 18-gauge needle in the intercoastal space.

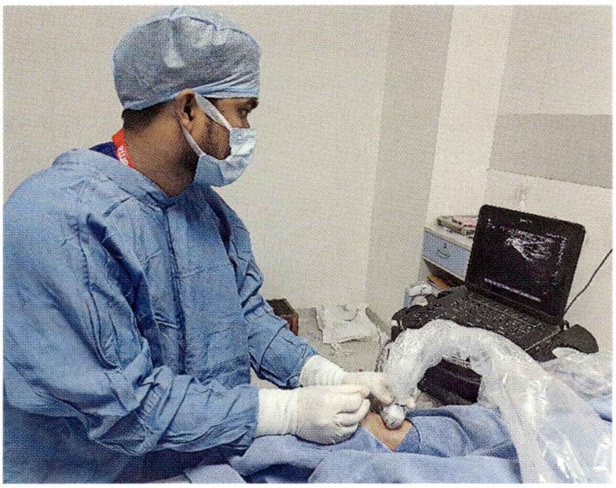

Fig. 6: Positioning and ergonomics for ultrasound (USG)-guided radial arterial cannulation (right hand).

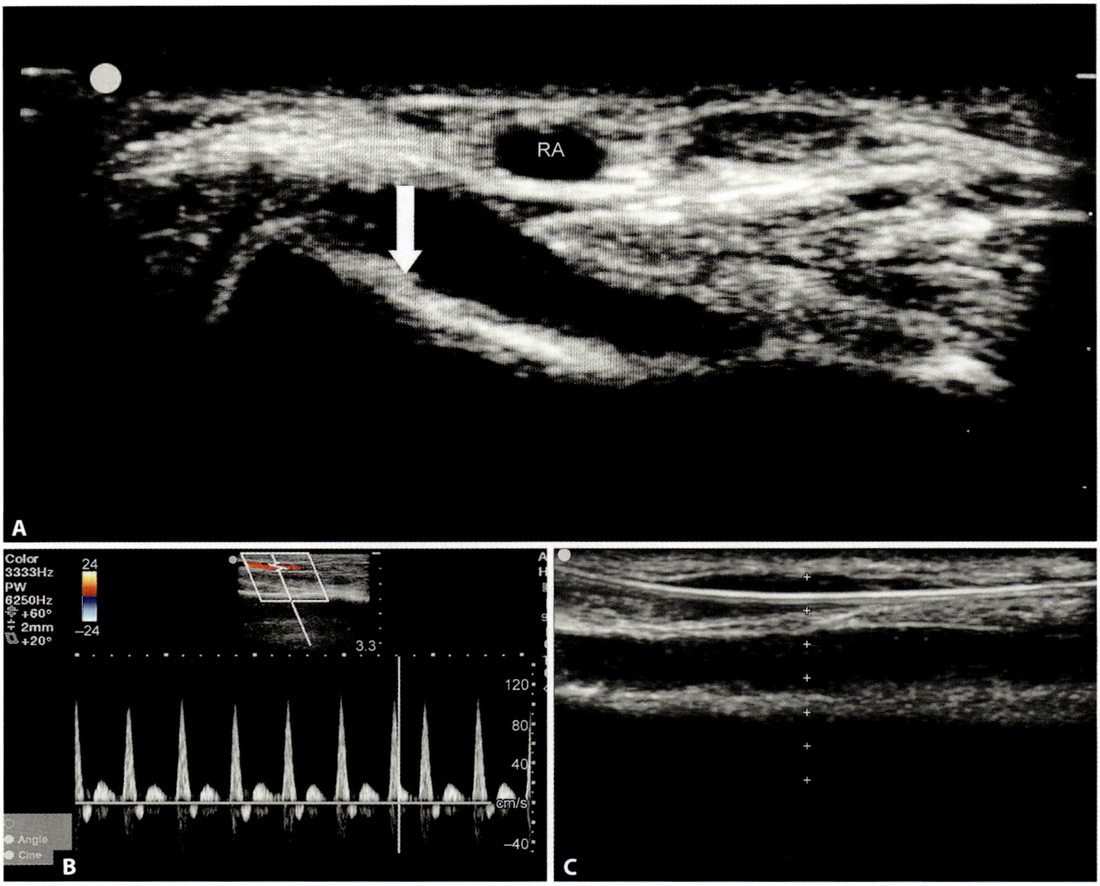

Figs. 7A to C: (A) Radial artery (RA) in transverse view; (B) RA in longitudinal view with pulse-wave Doppler confirming arterial waveform; (C) Arterial cannula in radial artery after insertion. (Arrow: radius bone)

Roll over the guidewire through the needle and remove the needle. Dilate the cavity using a dilator and insert an appropriate size pigtail depending upon the pathology like large size pigtail for abscess and hemothorax and fix it using suture.

Five key steps to perform ultrasound-guided thoracentesis ***(Figs. 9A and B)****:*

1. *Patient positioning and preparation:* Position the patient upright, leaning slightly forward with their arms supported on a table or chair to expose the back. If the patient cannot sit, a lateral decubitus position can be used. Perform hand hygiene, prepare the skin with an antiseptic solution, and drape the area for a sterile procedure.
2. *Ultrasound examination:* Use the ultrasound to locate the pleural effusion and identify a suitable site for needle insertion. The ideal site is at the midscapular line, above the diaphragm, and away from major vessels. Measure the depth of the fluid pocket and assess the surrounding structures, ensuring that the lung is not in the path of the needle.

3. *Marking the insertion site:* Once the appropriate site is identified, mark it with a sterile marker. The site should be selected where the pleural effusion is closest to the skin, ideally avoiding any intercostal vessels.
4. *Anesthesia and needle insertion:* Infiltrate local anesthesia at the site of puncture. Using the ultrasound as a guide, insert the thoracentesis needle at the marked site, angling it slightly upward toward the fluid pocket. Continuously monitor the needle's progress with ultrasound to ensure it enters the pleural space without puncturing the lung.
5. *Aspiration and fluid collection:* Once the needle is confirmed to be in the pleural space, attach a syringe or catheter to aspirate the fluid. Aspirate the required amount of fluid for diagnostic or therapeutic purposes, then remove the needle and apply a sterile dressing to the site. Monitor the patient for any immediate complications, such as pneumothorax.

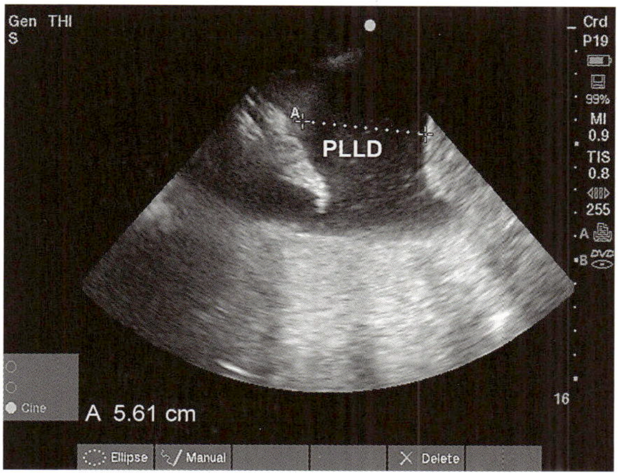

Fig. 8: Pleural line to lung distance (PLLD).

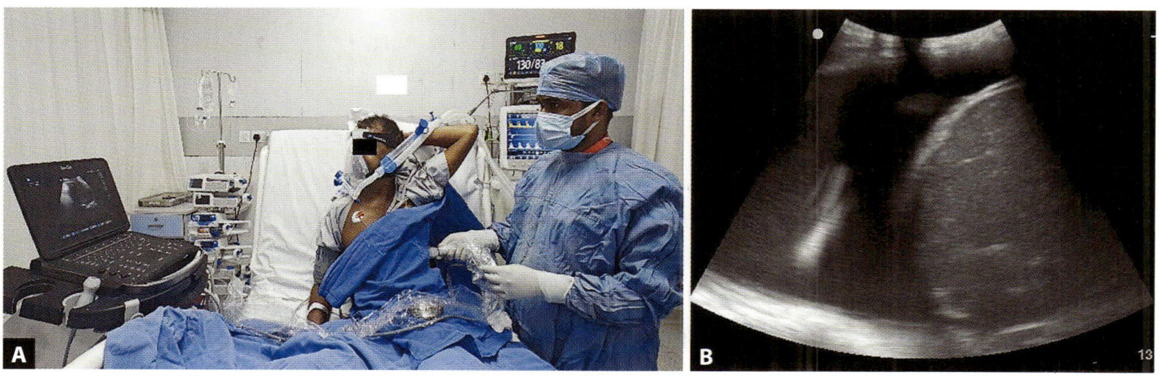

Figs. 9A and B: (A) Ergonomics for USG guided pleural tapping. Can also be done via posterior approach; (B) Intercostal drain visualized in pleural cavity.

PERICARDIOCENTESIS

- Pericardiocentesis is an emergency procedure used to remove excess fluid from the pericardial cavity, typically guided by a sonogram to ensure accurate needle placement.
- This condition, known as pericardial effusion, can arise from various causes, including congestive heart failure, pulmonary hypertension, infections such as tuberculosis, hypothyroidism, malignancies, trauma, and postmyocardial infarction. It may also occur after cardiac surgery due to surgical trauma, inflammatory responses, or changes in vascular permeability.
- Signs and symptoms of progressive pericardial effusion include muffled heart sounds during auscultation and fever, with some patients requiring vasopressors if they develop obstructive shock.
- Transthoracic echocardiography is crucial in diagnosing pericardial effusion, as it helps to determine the size, distribution, and hemodynamic impact of the fluid, guiding the pericardiocentesis procedure.[6]
- Since the fluid may not be uniformly distributed around the heart, multiple echocardiographic views are necessary to locate the area of maximal accumulation and to plan the safest and most effective approach for fluid removal.

Five key steps to perform ultrasound-guided pericardiocentesis:

1. *Patient positioning and preparation:* Position the patient in a semirecumbent or supine position with the head elevated to 30–45°. This helps to bring the pericardial effusion to the most accessible area. Ensure proper hand hygiene and use sterile techniques, including draping the area to maintain a sterile field.
2. *Ultrasound examination:* Use transthoracic ultrasound to identify the pericardial effusion. The subxiphoid, parasternal, or apical views are commonly used. Determine the largest and safest area for needle insertion by assessing the size and location of the effusion. Measure the distance from the skin to the pericardial fluid to gauge the depth of needle insertion.
3. *Marking the insertion site:* Once the optimal site is identified, mark it on the skin. The subxiphoid approach is most commonly used, but the choice depends on where the effusion is most accessible and the patient's anatomy.
4. *Needle insertion and aspiration:* After administering local anesthesia at the marked site, insert the needle at the appropriate angle under continuous ultrasound guidance. Advance the needle carefully toward the effusion, constantly monitoring its position on the ultrasound screen. Once the needle tip is in the pericardial space, withdraw fluid slowly to relieve the pressure around the heart **(Figs. 10A and B)**.
5. *Postprocedure monitoring:* After aspirating the pericardial fluid, remove the needle and apply a sterile dressing to the site. Continue to monitor the patient closely for any signs of complications, such as recurrent effusion, infection, or injury to surrounding structures. A follow-up ultrasound may be performed to ensure the effusion has been adequately drained.

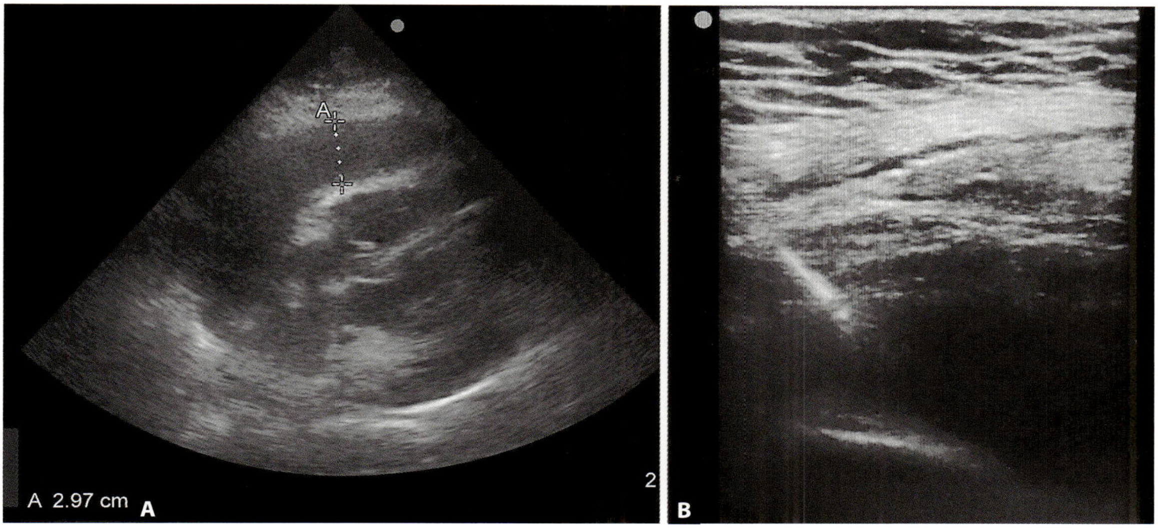

Figs. 10A and B: (A) Pericardial effusion in subxiphoid view with Echo probe; (B) Catheter in place for pericardiocentesis with the help of straight vascular probe.

FUTURE DIRECTIONS

- The increasing availability of portable USG devices is expected to change scenarios in remote and urgent care settings. As workloads increase, innovations such as cloud-based data management for USG images are being introduced, offering streamlined solutions for documentation and analysis.
- One exciting development is the use of POCUS combined with machine learning algorithms to accelerate patient triage through image pattern recognition. This approach is likely to lead to automated USG image interpretation, which could revolutionize emergency care by providing quicker and more objective diagnoses.
- Additionally, the exploration of augmented and virtual reality applications for USG is paving the way for more advanced educational tools and training methods.

CONCLUSION

- The use of USG for procedural guidance has significantly improved safety and success rates in emergency interventions. Procedures such as vascular access, thoracentesis, and pericardiocentesis benefit from enhanced precision, reducing complications and improving patient comfort.
- The portability and ease of use of modern USG devices enable their application in resource-limited settings, including prehospital care and disaster management scenarios, further extending their utility.

REFERENCES

1. Rosenblatt WH, Yanez ND. A decision tree approach to airway management pathways in the 2022 difficult airway algorithm of the American society of anesthesiologists. Anesth. Analg. 2022;134(5):910-5.
2. Watanabe H, Nakazawa H, Tokumine J, Yorozu T. Real-time vs. static ultrasound-guided needle cricothyroidotomy: a randomized crossover simulation trial. Sci Rep. 2025;15(1):8112.
3. Elshikh ST, Thomas B, Taha M, Shaikh AM, Alkhazendar AH, Awan M, et al. Evaluating the Accuracy of Point-of-Care Ultrasound for Peripheral Intravenous Cannulation in Emergency and Trauma Patients: A Systematic Review. Cureus. 2025;17(5):e83625.
4. Wang A, Hendin A, Millington SJ, Koenig S, Eisen LA, Shiloh AL. Better with Ultrasound: Arterial Line Placement. Chest. 2020;157(3):574-9.
5. Hassan M, Touman AA, Grabczak EM, Skaarup SH, Faber K, Blyth KG, et al. Imaging of pleural disease. Breathe (Sheff). 2024;20(1):230172.
6. Jung HO. Pericardial effusion and pericardiocentesis: role of echocardiography. Korean Circ J. 2012;42(11):725-34.

CHAPTER 10

Ultrasound in Cardiac Arrest

Asif Dabeer Jafri, Utsav Anand Mani, Alka Verma, Divya Srivastava

WHAT YOU WILL LEARN IN THIS CHAPTER?

A. Understand the rationale for incorporating ultrasound into cardiac arrest management

B. Examine various protocols and practical considerations for implementing ultrasound during cardiac arrest

INTRODUCTION

Various medical societies advocate for use of point-of-care ultrasound (POCUS), deeming it a vital aspect of training for emergency and critical care physicians. Current guidelines suggest that ultrasound should be utilized as an adjunctive diagnostic tool when there is a clinical suspicion of a specific reversible cause, provided it is conducted by skilled personnel without interrupting cardiopulmonary resuscitation (CPR).[1,2]

WHY ULTRASOUND IN CARDIOPULMONARY RESUSCITATION?

Point-of-care ultrasound serves as an essential instrument during cardiac arrest situations, as it can detect both reversible causes of the condition and the presence or absence of cardiac activity.[3] Patients experiencing cardiac arrest often exhibit significant shock, resulting in weak pulses that are challenging to palpate. In cases where patients are assessed to have no pulse upon palpation, ultrasound may reveal evidence of cardiac activity.[4,5] In such scenarios, POCUS provides a more accurate assessment of cardiac function, potentially preventing unnecessary CPR and thereby reducing the risk of further trauma to the patient.

The absence of cardiac activity on ultrasound during cardiac arrest is a strong predictor of poor survival outcomes. In the REASON trial of 793 patients with pulseless electrical activity (PEA) and asystole, 33% showed initial cardiac activity on ultrasound, while 67% did not. Among those with detected cardiac activity, >50% successfully achieved return of spontaneous circulation (ROSC), resulting in enhanced survival rates for both hospital admission and discharge. Further analysis of this trial stratified patients with PEA and asystole based on their initial cardiac activity on ultrasound, categorizing it as either "organized" or "disorganized" activity. The findings revealed that the use of adrenergic agents in patients with organized cardiac activity was associated with improved survival compared to those with disorganized activity.[6] This suggests that POCUS may play a crucial role in identifying subsets of patients with PEA and asystole who exhibit different responses to resuscitation, thereby guiding more tailored and effective management strategies.

The updated guidelines have emphasized minimizing interruptions during ongoing CPR and using audiovisual feedback for assessing ongoing CPR performance. Further, it has been advised to consider the use of ultrasound during cardiac arrest to determine the underlying cause of arrest.

ULTRASOUND IN THE DIAGNOSTIC EVALUATION AND MANAGEMENT OF CARDIAC ARREST

In the context of CPR, it is essential to evaluate the reversible causes of cardiac arrest, which are summarized by the 5H and 5T categories as per the American Heart Association (AHA) algorithm, as illustrated in **Table 1**. Ultrasound may be utilized for diagnosis in cases indicated with an asterisk (*).

In the course of resuscitation, ultrasound examination facilitates the swift identification of the root cause of cardiac arrest, enabling the prompt implementation of targeted and effective intervention strategies, as demonstrated in **Table 2**. The patient's medical history frequently offers insights into possible poisoning or toxin exposure. Furthermore, arterial blood gas analysis plays a crucial role in assessing hypoxia, electrolyte disturbances (such as hypo- or hyperkalemia), and metabolic acidosis.

Various Echocardiographic (Echo) Protocols in Cardiac Arrest are Given Here

The First Echo Protocol in Cardiac Arrest is EASy-ALS Protocol

Introduced in 2020, the EASy-ALS protocol (Echocardiographic Assessment using Subcostal-only view in Advanced Life Support) aims to incorporate ultrasound into resuscitation efforts while reducing interruptions to chest compressions.[7] The step-by-step guide (steps 1 to 4) is outlined below, with the corresponding algorithm presented in **Figure 1**.

1. *Preparation during cardiopulmonary resuscitation before pulse/rhythm check*
   - Wait until the current 2-minute cycle of chest compressions is completed.
   - Remove any obstacles to the ultrasound, such as clothing or dressings
   - Place the ultrasound probe on the patient to obtain a subcostal four-chamber view (steps written below).
2. *During pulse/rhythm check*
   - Perform the subcostal four-chamber ultrasound view and record the images quickly
   - Resuming chest compressions within 10 seconds.

TABLE 1: Reversible causes of cardiac arrest 5H and 5T.

5H	*5T*
Hypovolemia*	Thrombosis (pulmonary)*
Hypoxia	Thrombosis (myocardial infarction)*
Hydrogen ions (acidosis)	Tamponade (cardiac)*
Hyper-/hypokalemia	Tension pneumothorax*
Hypovolemia	Toxins

TABLE 2: USG findings during cardiac arrest and its clinical applications.

Cause	*USG findings*	*Implications*
Cardiac tamponade	Pericardial effusion with ventricular collapse	Pericardiocentesis
Tension pneumothorax	Absent lung sliding	Immediate decompression
Massive pulmonary embolism	Right ventricular dilation and McConnell's sign	Thrombolysis
Hypovolemia	Collapsed IVC; reduced cardiac filling	Fluid resuscitation
Pseudo-PEA	Cardiac motion in the absence of pulses	Vasopressors and fluids

(IVC: inferior vena cava; PEA: pulseless electrical activity; USG: ultrasound)

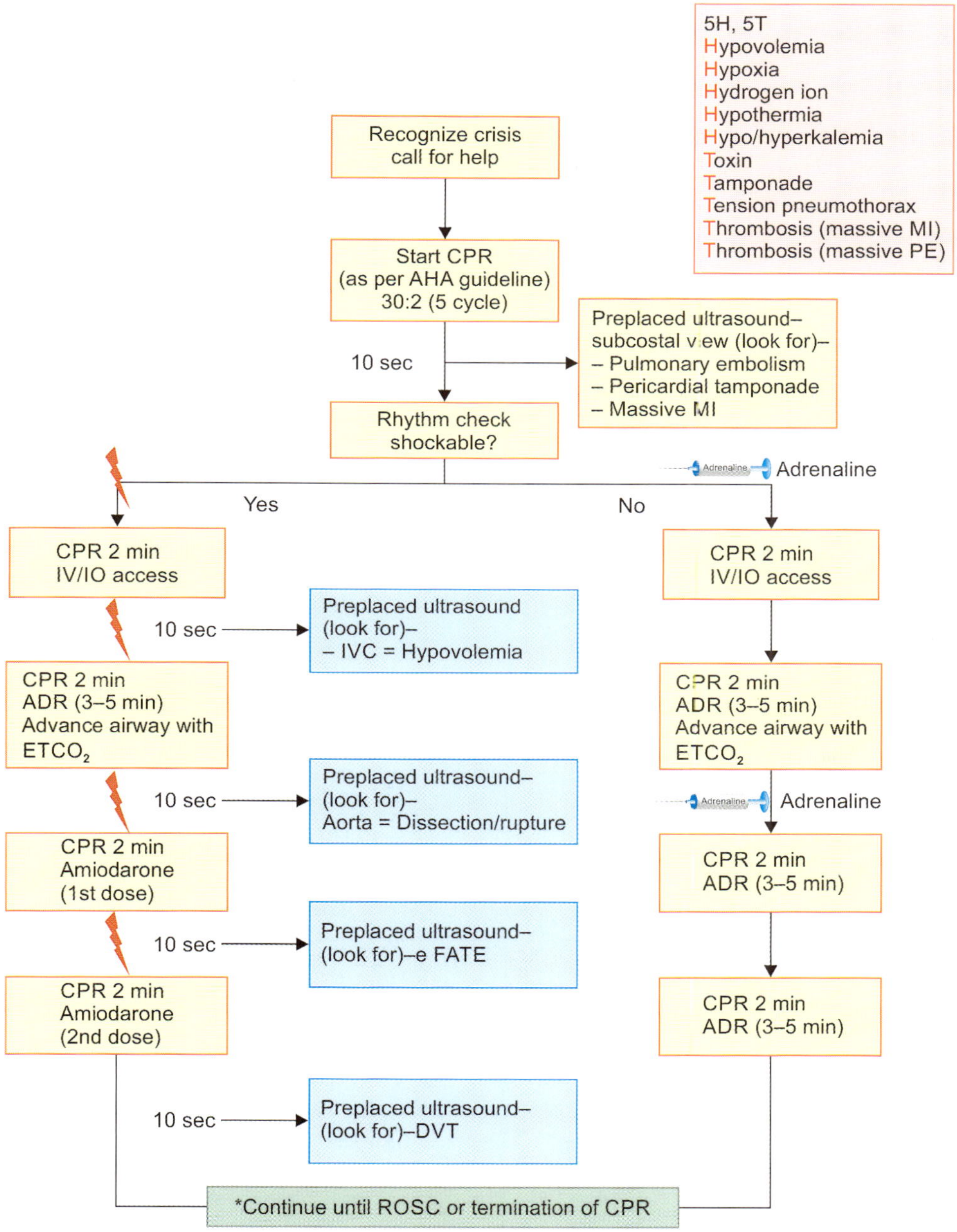

Fig. 1: Ultrasound (USG) incorporated in cardiopulmonary resuscitation (CPR) algorithm.

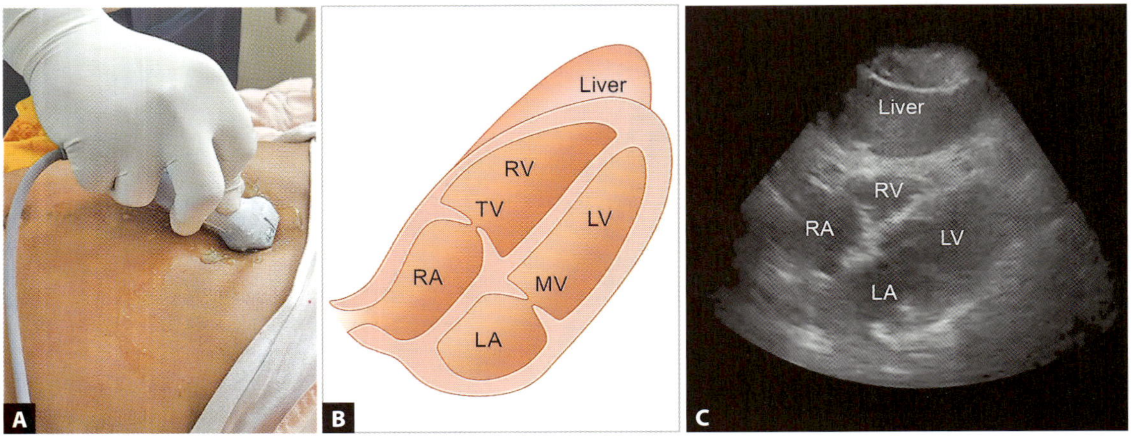

Figs. 2A to C: Obtaining a subcostal four-chamber view; (A) Probe positioning; (B) Schematic diagram of subcostal view; (C) USG picture of subcostal view. (LA: left atrium; LV: left ventricle; RA: right atrium; RV: right ventricle; USG: ultrasound)

3. *After pulse/rhythm check*
   - Interpret the recorded ultrasound images immediately
   - Communicate findings with the team leader
   - Determine if additional focused or lung ultrasound is needed in subsequent pulse checks.
4. *Additional evaluations anytime during cardiopulmonary resuscitation but preferably not during compressions*
   - Assess the inferior vena cava (IVC) to estimate right-sided filling pressure
   - Check the aorta for signs of aneurysm, dissection, or rupture
   - Confirm correct airway placement and check for esophageal intubation
   - Scan the chest for pneumothorax and pleural effusion
   - Assess the abdomen for any intraperitoneal bleeding
   - Evaluate deep veins of the leg for signs of thrombosis.

Obtaining the subcostal four-chamber view (refer to ***Figure 2A to C*** *):* To acquire an optimal subcostal four-chamber view, follow these steps.

1. *Select the appropriate probe:* Use a phased array probe for better penetration and image clarity.
2. *Adjust the depth:* Set the ultrasound depth between 16 and 24 cm to ensure adequate visualization.
3. *Position the patient:* Have the patient lie supine, flex the knees, and take a deep inspiration to bring the heart closer to the probe.
4. *Probe placement:* Position the probe just below the xiphoid process with gentle pressure.
5. *Probe orientation:* Align the probe marker toward the left shoulder (approximately at 3 o'clock position) to obtain the correct cardiac axis.
6. *Image acquisition:* Ensure that all four chambers of the heart, along with the tricuspid and mitral valves, are clearly visualized.

The Second Echocardiographic Approach in Cardiac Arrest is the SESAME Protocol

SESAME protocol: Proposed in 2015, the SESAME protocol (Sequential Echocardiographic Scanning Assessing Mechanism or Origin of Severe Shock of

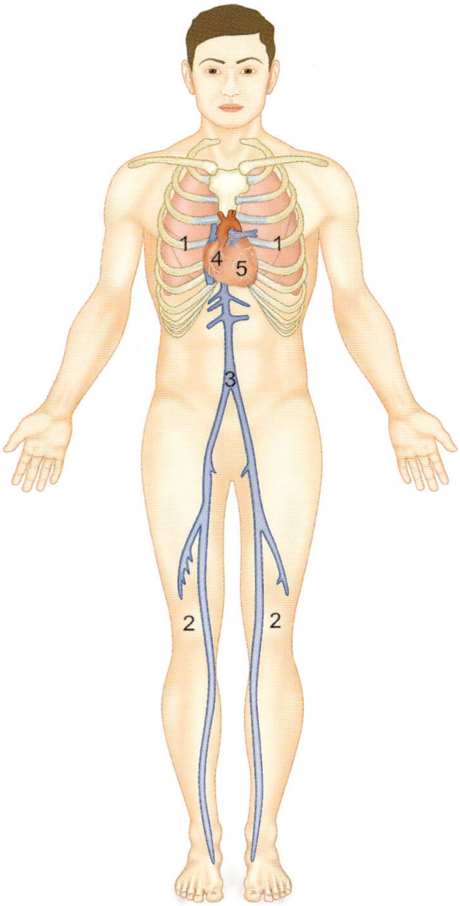

Fig. 3: Probe positions in SESAME protocol. (SESAME: Sequential Echocardiographic Scanning Assessing Mechanism or Origin of Severe Shock of Indistinct Cause)

Indistinct Cause) provides a structured, stepwise ultrasound assessment during cardiac arrest.[8] This protocol prioritizes scanning in an order that minimizes disruption to chest compressions. The different probe position in this protocol is shown in **Figure 3**.

Scanning sequence:

1. *Lungs:* Assess for pneumothorax, pleural effusion, or pulmonary edema.
2. *Legs:* Evaluate for deep vein thrombosis (DVT) as a potential source of pulmonary embolism.
3. *Belly:* Check for intra-abdominal bleeding or free fluid.
4. *Pericardium:* Detect pericardial effusion or tamponade (can be done during compressions).
5. *Heart:* Assess cardiac motion, chamber size, and overall function.

Limitations and considerations:

- The protocol requires switching between multiple probes (linear, abdominal, and cardiac), which may be time-consuming.
- This challenge can be mitigated by using a 5 MHz microconvex probe, if available, to streamline the assessment.
- Chest compressions should only be paused during lung and heart examinations (first and last steps), while pericardial assessment can be performed during ongoing compressions.

The Third Protocol is SHoC (Sonography in Hypotension and Cardiac Arrest) Protocol

This protocol was endorsed by the International Federation for Emergency Medicine (IFEM) in 2017 as a standardized ultrasound method for the assessment of undifferentiated shock and cardiac arrest within the field of emergency medicine.[9] This protocol comprises two primary pathways:

1. *SHoC hypotension:* Aimed at evaluating patients experiencing shock to distinguish between cardiogenic and noncardiogenic origins.
2. *SHoC cardiac arrest:* A targeted strategy for assessing cardiac function and identifying reversible causes during resuscitation efforts.

   The SHoC cardiac arrest protocol is composed of core views, supplementary views, and additional views, all of which deliver essential diagnostic insights while minimally interfering with CPR procedures.

- *Core views (performed in all patients):* These essential views focus on cardiac function and structure.
    - Cardiac (subxiphoid or parasternal long-axis view)
    - *Fluid:* Presence of pericardial effusion or tamponade
    - *Form:* Chamber size and shape (e.g., small or dilated ventricles)
    - Is there right heart strain based on the right-to-left ventricular size ratio?
    - *Function:* Assessment of ventricular contractility
    - Are the heart valves opening properly?
    - Is there adequate blood flow?
- *Supplementary views:* These views provide further assessment of lung and vascular status.
    - Lung (bilateral anterior and lateral views)
    - Is lung sliding present?
    - Are B-lines visible? (bilateral or focal).
    - Is there pleural effusion or fluid accumulation?
    - IVC (subxiphoid or transhepatic view)
    - What is the IVC diameter?
    - Is there respiratory variation in size?
- *Additional views (performed based on clinical indication):*
    - *Abdominal and pelvic views:* Evaluate for free fluid or hemorrhage
    - *Aortic view:* Check for abdominal aortic aneurysm (AAA)
    - *DVT view:* Assess for proximal iliofemoral thrombosis
    - *Airway view:* Detect esophageal intubation (double tract sign)

SHoC protocol for hypotension: This protocol follows a tiered approach.[10]

- *Core views:* Identify the type of shock (cardiogenic vs. noncardiogenic) using
    - Basic cardiac views (subxiphoid or parasternal long-axis) to assess pericardial fluid, structure, and ventricular function
    - Lung views to check for pleural fluid and B-lines, indicating fluid status
    - IVC views to assess volume responsiveness
- *Supplementary views:* Expanded cardiac assessments, including parasternal and apical windows to refine evaluation of cardiac form and function
- *Additional views:* Used when clinically necessary, including scans for AAA, pelvic free fluid, DVT, and airway integrity.

Key advantages of the SHoC protocol:

- Provides a systematic approach to ultrasound in critically ill patients
- Helps to differentiate between cardiogenic and noncardiogenic shock
- Identifies reversible causes of cardiac arrest with minimal CPR interruptions
- Can be tailored based on clinical urgency and available time.

Additional echocardiographic protocols utilized in cardiac arrest scenarios are outlined in **Table 3**.

PRACTICAL CONSIDERATIONS

While multiple protocols guide ultrasound assessment during cardiac arrest, certain key practices have proven effective in real-world scenarios.[16,17]

- *Prioritize chest compressions:* Ensure that ultrasound use does not disrupt high-quality CPR.
- *Prepare in advance:* Position the probe and resuscitation team before a scheduled CPR pause. Activate clip recording with sufficient duration to capture relevant findings.
- *Keep it brief:* Acquire cardiac images quickly during pulse or rhythm checks (within

TABLE 3: Ultrasound (USG) protocols during cardiac arrest.

No.	Protocol	Published	Focus
1	*FEER:*[11] Focused Echocardiographic Evaluation in Resuscitation	2007	Focus only on the heart
2	*CAUSE:*[12] Cardiac Arrest Ultrasound Exam	2007	Focus on heart and lungs
3	*FEEL:*[13] Focused Echocardiographic Entry Level	2009	Focus only on the heart
4	*CASA:*[14] Cardiac Arrest Sonographic Assessment	2018	Focus on the heart, lungs, and abdomen
5	*PEA:*[15] Pulmonary, Epigastric, and Abdominal Scan	2010	Focus on heart, lungs, abdomen, and vascular ultrasound

10 seconds), postponing interpretation to avoid delays.

- *Resume CPR promptly:* Immediately restart compressions before interpreting the recorded images. Additional ultrasound assessments (e.g., lungs, abdomen, and vascular structures) can be conducted during ongoing CPR when feasible.
- *Communicate findings clearly:* Share ultrasound results with the team to guide further resuscitation efforts.

CONCLUSION

The incorporation of ultrasound into the management of cardiac arrest has revolutionized resuscitation practices by enhancing diagnostic precision and improving patient outcomes. Various protocols, such as EASy-ALS, SESAME, and SHoC, offer systematic approaches for the effective use of ultrasound while minimizing disruptions to CPR. By facilitating real-time evaluations of cardiac contractility, perfusion status, and reversible causes, ultrasound acts as a vital tool in informing clinical decisions. Nevertheless, its application must be carefully managed to prevent delays in chest compressions, highlighting the importance of adequate training and adherence to established best practices. As technology and expertise advances, the significance of ultrasound in resuscitation is poised to grow, bridging the divide between sophisticated diagnostics and prompt, lifesaving actions.

REFERENCES

1. Soar J, Böttiger BW, Carli P, Couper K, Deakin CD, Djärv T, et al. European Resuscitation Council Guidelines 2021: Adult advanced life support. Resuscitation. 2021;161:115-51.
2. Merchant RM, Topjian AA, Panchal AR, Cheng A, Aziz K, Berg KM, et al. Part 1: Executive Summary: 2020 American Heart Association Guidelines for Cardiopulmonary Resuscitation and Emergency Cardiovascular Care. Circulation. 2020;142:S337-S357.
3. Gaspari R, Weekes A, Adhikari S, Noble VE, Nomura JT, Theodoro D, et al. Emergency department point-of-care ultrasound in out-of-hospital and in-ED cardiac arrest. Resuscitation. 2016;109:33-9.
4. Salen P, Melniker L, Chooljian C, Rose JS, Alteveer J, Reed J, et al. Does the presence or absence of sonographically identified cardiac activity predict resuscitation outcomes of cardiac arrest patients? Am J Emerg Med. 2005;23:459-62.
5. Zengin S, Gümüşboğa H, Sabak M, Eren ŞH, Altunbas G, Al B. Comparison of manual pulse palpation, cardiac ultrasonography and Doppler ultrasonography to check the pulse in cardiopulmonary arrest patients. Resuscitation. 2018;133:59-64.
6. Gaspari R, Weekes A, Adhikari S, Noble V, Nomura JT, Theodoro D, et al. A retrospective study of pulseless electrical activity, bedside ultrasound identifies interventions during resuscitation associated with improved survival to hospital

admission. A REASON Study. Resuscitation. 2017;120:103-7.

7. Bughrara N, Herrick SL, Leimer E, Sirigaddi K, Roberts K, Pustavoitau A. Focused cardiac ultrasound and the periresuscitative period: a case series of resident-performed echocardiographic assessment using subcostal-only view in advanced life support. A A Pract. 2020;14(10):e01278.
8. Lichtenstein D, Malbrain M. Critical care ultrasound in cardiac arrest. Technological requirements for performing the SESAME-protocol—a holistic approach. Anestezjologia Intensywna Terapia. 2015;47(5):487-97.
9. Atkinson P, Bowra J, Milne J, Lewis D, Lambert M, Jarman B, et al. International Federation for Emergency Medicine Consensus Statement: Sonography in hypotension and cardiac arrest (SHoC): An international consensus on the use of point of care ultrasound for undifferentiated hypotension and during cardiac arrest. Can J Emerg Med. 2017;19(6):459-70.
10. Atkinson P, Bowra J, Milne J, Lambert M, Jarman B, Noble V, et al. LO042: Sonography in Hypotension and Cardiac Arrest (SHoC)-Hypotension: Derivation of an evidence-based consensus algorithm for the integration of point of care ultrasound into resuscitation of hypotensive patients. Can J Emerg Med. 2016;18(S1):S44-44.
11. Breitkreutz R, Walcher F, Seeger FH. Focused echocardiographic evaluation in resuscitation management: Concept of an advanced life support–conformed algorithm. Crit Care Med. 2007;35(5):S150-61.
12. Hernandez C, Shuler K, Hannan H, Sonyika C, Likourezos A, Marshall J. C.A.U.S.E.: Cardiac arrest ultra-sound exam—a better approach to managing patients in primary non-arrhythmogenic cardiac arrest. Resuscitation. 2008;76(2):198-206.
13. Breitkreutz R, Walcher F, Ilper H, Seeger FH, Price S, Via G, et al. Focused echocardiography in life support: the subcostal window: what the surgeon should know for critical care applications. Eur J Trauma Emerg Surg. 2009;35(4):347.
14. Clattenburg EJ, Wroe PC, Gardner K, Schultz C, Gelber J, Singh A, et al. Implementation of the Cardiac Arrest Sonographic Assessment (CASA) protocol for patients with cardiac arrest is associated with shorter CPR pulse checks. Resuscitation. 2018;131:69-73.
15. Testa A, Cibinel GA, Portale G, Forte P, Giannuzzi R, Pignataro G, et al. The proposal of an integrated ultrasonographic approach into the ALS algorithm for cardiac arrest: the PEA protocol. Eur Rev Med Pharmacol Sci. 2010;14(2):77-88.
16. Paul JA, Panzer OP. Point-of-care ultrasound in cardiac arrest. Anesthesiology. 2021; 135(3):508-19.
17. Magon F, Longhitano Y, Savioli G, Piccioni A, Tesauro M, Del Duca F, et al. Point-of-Care Ultrasound (POCUS) in Adult Cardiac Arrest: Clinical Review. Diagnostics (Basel). 2024; 14(4):434.

Index

Page numbers followed by *f* refer to figure and *t* refer to table.